RAPID WEIGHT LOSS HYPNOSIS:

A GUIDED MEDITATION TO STOP EMOTIONAL EATING WITH IMPRESSIVE AFFIRMATION. FOR WOMEN WHO WANT TO BURN FAT, CONQUER SELF-ESTEEM, AND HEAL THEIR BODIES.

AUTHOR:

Samantha Clooney

Table of Contents

Introduction

"I know I can do anything I set my mind to because I am strong and confident." Affirmations like this one are intended to lift a person's spirits when feeling low or anxious. Claims can be about anything and are relatively easy to think of so long as they are positive. When you say this statement to yourself, "I am perfect just the way that I am," you don't have to believe it is necessary, but they are vital for personal growth. It has been proven that people who tell themselves at least one good thing (whether they believe that statement or not) have less stressful days and are generally happier than those who don't. Positive reinforcement is absolutely essential for the purpose of losing weight because those who struggle with their weight usually feel overwhelmed, stressed, depressed, or believe that they are unworthy. With this type of mindset, it's no wonder you're unhappy with your weight. There are so many things in life that can bring you down, but your own body weight doesn't need to be one of them.

When people are upset, they will often starve themselves or eat comfort food to feel better. You probably purchased this book because you realized that you're in an unhealthy cycle. First, you may have had something happen to you during the day that has stressed you out, which you will then ruminate and obsess over how ugly you think you are. Negative thoughts lead to poor self-image and low self-esteem, which can make anyone depressed or angry. So, the following (unhealthy) step is usually grabbing a slice of cake, a bag of chips, a chocolate brownie, or other junk food to make you feel better. While you're eating it, you feel better, but then afterward, you realize you may have gone too far and start to feel ashamed, embarrassed, or even guilty. These feelings then trigger another emotional response, which stresses you out, and here we are back at the beginning again. It is a vicious, unending circle.

This book will help you control your mindset by feeling uplifted and confident about developing positive habits to healthy eating and regular exercise. Don't think that meditation alone will decrease your weight because there are other things that you can do to continue taking the pounds off to reach your ideal body weight. However, reading this book of meditation, affirmations, and hypnosis will help you become motivated to lose the pounds as if they were never a problem in the first place. The core issue here is that your brain is stuck in this negative cycle, one of the leading causes of binge eating and intuitive eating. Have you ever noticed that you feel sluggish and have low energy when you eat many carbs and processed foods? That's because those foods have nothing good in them. The idea of hypnosis is to bring you to a subconscious state and trick your mind, so you don't feel a certain way, and the affirmations are to help build your self-esteem, so you feel like getting up and walking or going for a run - maybe you'll be inspired to grab a gym membership. Meditation is used to help you relax and train your mind not to think negatively, so you can better focus on your goals ahead.

Throughout the meditations in this book, I promise that you will be well on your way to success and become motivated to reach your desired body weight. Remember, you don't have to be perfect to complete your goals; as long as you are always trying, you will succeed. Throughout this book, make sure that you lie flat on a comfortable surface or naturally sit in a comfortable chair. Also, try to avoid stressful environments, such as a workspace or office, a place with noisy pets, children, or other people in general. The goal before starting each exercise is to have your mind clear so that these exercises can work. Bring only positive energy into your being and listen carefully to the meditations.

Chapter 1   What is Hypnosis?

One from the year 4000 BC, derived cuneiform about suggestion is that the Priest doctors already practiced a preform of the present hypnosis in a healthy sleep was produced through particular instructions.

Other traditions include thousands of years old Greek writings, Egyptian hieroglyphs, and mentions in the Mahabharata of the Hindus. In India, for example, hypnosis has been divided into three stages: "sleep awake" and "dream sleep."

Nowadays, these techniques are used in the form of self-hypnosis in advanced yoga practices, which can cause significant physiological changes. In ancient Egypt, similar methods were also practiced very early on.

Priests, who at the same time served as doctors of the people, led a state of hypnosis by the still standard fixation method by holding sickly shiny metal discs in front of their eyes. By laying on of hands combined with healing suggestions, then the recovery should be encouraged.

The Greek and Egyptian sleeping temples are mainly well known in which the sick were put into several days of restorative sleep. Supported by whispered suggestions from the priests, great healing successes were achieved.

The hypnosis as a ritual of temple sleep can continue until 400 BC. We traced back over 1,000 years to Greece, Rome, Egypt, and Carthage. Hand paralyzes, blindness, and skin diseases were treated.

The use of hypnosis has a long tradition, even among shamans from various cultures. They have long been using the positive effects of hypnoses-like techniques such as drum rhythms to put patients in a trance state where the unconscious is more amenable to healing.

In 1890, natives in British Guiana were reported to heal headaches with the help of hypnotic sleep. Even today, American Indians enter into a trance state through rhythmic dances, and Australian medicine men use hypnosis during initiation rites.

Already in the 11th-century, members of a monastic order practiced self-hypnosis using fixation on their own center. The physician Theophrastus Bombastus von Hohenheim (1493-1541), also called Paracelsus, recognized the curative effect of positive suggestions and recommended hypnosis, especially in nervous diseases.

Their partially bad reputation received this healing method during the Inquisition. The Inquisitors declared it a "devil's work" in modern times and did not follow church-thinking and acting people, whereby the hypnosis fell into oblivion.

However, numerous delinquents have also been reported during this period, self-suggesting pain relief during a torture procedure to become immune to the torments.

The healing effects of hypnotic practices have been attributed to superhuman forces, mostly gods, mediated by a human medium from antiquity to the Middle Ages.

On the other hand, the German physician Franz Anton Mesmer (1734-1815), regarded as the "godfather of modern hypnosis," viewed hypnosis not from a mystical-religious but a scientific point of view.

For him, the healings of Gassner were not supernatural, but he classified hypnosis as a natural force localized outside of man. It was the beginning of a new era of this healing method.

Mesmer set up the theory of animal magnetism because he believed that every human being possessed a universal fluid that would be distributed unequally in the body during illnesses.

One could cancel this imbalance by magnetic healing currents, which he wanted to achieve by laying on hands, air strokes, or vessels with magnetized liquids.

In his group treatments, several people were sitting around a barrel of water filled with iron bars sticking out to touch the sick. In keeping with the spirit of the times (according to Volta, Newton, and Galvani), he wanted to substantiate the hypnotic phenomena physically by the power of magnetism.

When he became well-known, the process of hypnotizing was also called "Mesmerizing" (in English, the verb "to mesmerize" is still used today). Mesmer himself practiced as a fashion doctor, among others, at the French court, where he treated the Queen Marie-Antoinette and the Mozart family.

However, since he did not induce hypnotic sleep, it is questionable whether he can be called a hypnotist. Instead, he used an opposite psychological phenomenon called "healing crisis," The patients were put into a temporary state of hysteria. Although he had many followers, he ultimately could not have his method accredited to the Academy of Sciences in Paris. Although he later withdrew this assumption when he realized that the trance state is different from sleep, the term hypnosis had already prevailed at this time.

Mesmer was also the first to perform eye surgery under hypnosis, triggering a discussion about new applications and treatment options. Before introducing anesthetics such as ether, nitrous oxide, and chloroform, hypnosis was an essential technique for pain-free surgical procedures.

However, after the discovery of these anesthetics, it was forgotten as an anesthetic option. But the fairs saw a career: showpeople found amusing the audience by making people ridicule themselves in hypnosis.

The American psychiatrist and psychotherapist Milton H. Ericksons (1901-1980) helped the hypnosis with his research results and publications ultimately in Germany to a rebirth.

He enriched the therapeutic intervention inventory with his hypnotherapeutic approaches, making modern hypnotherapy more popular in the last 25 years.

When he fell ill with polio at the age of 18, he spent the time of his recovery using imagination training and visualization exercises to train his muscles to walk with crutches after just one year. The results of his mental activities fascinated him so much that he began to engage in hypnosis and soon developed new techniques.

He tested this after completing his medical studies during the treatments and curing several patients who had failed other therapies.

Above all, Erickson used metaphors to activate new or buried resources in the patient. His indirect and permissive suggestions contrasted with the hitherto prevailing authoritarian style and revolutionized therapeutic hypnosis.

In 2006, hypnotherapy was scientifically recognized by the Scientific Advisory Council on Psychotherapy. Hypnosis research has evolved significantly in the last 20 years. In ancient and medieval times, hypnosis may have been like magic, but today there are scientific explanations for the brain processes that occur during a trance state.

In clinical studies, the effectiveness of hypnosis in medicine, for example, in the physiological influence of the immune system, has been demonstrated.

There are a variety of therapy schools today that teach a variety of hypnotic approaches. Due to the current trend towards natural healing methods, the interest in hypnotherapy is growing steadily.

In reality, it is sometimes difficult to distinguish what is scientifically proven and what is not. For example, we know that psychology can help us lose weight, but we don't know much about other somewhat more confusing methods, such as hypnosis.

Is it possible that hypnosis helps us lose weight? Next, we analyze how they use hypnotherapy in different clinics that offer weight loss and what the scientific research says about it.

Chapter 2   Which Methods exist?

There are several self-hypnosis techniques; however, they are all based on one concept: focusing on a single idea, object, image, or word. It is the key that opens the door to trance. You can achieve focus in many ways, so there are so many different techniques that can be applied. After a period of initial learning, those who have learned a method, and have continued to practice it, realize that they can skip specific steps. In this part, we will take a look at the essential self-hypnosis techniques.

The Betty Erickson Method

Here I'll summarize the most practical points of this method of Betty Erickson, wife of Milton Erickson, the most famous hypnotist of 1900.

Choose something you don't like about yourself. Turn it into an image, and then turn this image into a positive one. If you don't want your body shape, take a picture of your body, then turn it into a snapshot of your beautiful self with a body you would like to have. Before inducing self-hypnosis, give yourself a time limit before hypnotizing yourself mentally or, better yet, saying aloud the following sentence, "I induce self-hypnosis for X minutes." Your mind will take time like a Swiss watch.

How do you practice?

Take three objects around you, preferably small and bright, like a door handle, a light spot on a painting, etc., and fix your attention on each one of them. Take three sounds from your environment, traffic, fridge noise, etc., and set your attention on each one. Take three sensations you are feeling, the itchy nose, tingling in the leg, the feeling of air passing through the nose, etc. It's better to use unusual sensations, such as the sensation of the right foot inside the shoe, to which attention is not usually drawn. Don't fix your attention for too long, just enough to make you aware of what you see, feel, or try. The mind is quick. Then, in the same way, switch to two objects, two sounds, two sensations. Always be calm while switching to an object, a sound, a feeling. If you have done things correctly, you are in a trance, ready for the next step.

Now let your mind wander, as you did in class when the teacher spoke and you looked out of the window, and you were in another place, in another time, in another space, in a place where you would have liked to be, so completely forget about everything else. Now recall the initial image. Perhaps the mind wanders, from time to time, it gets distracted, maybe it goes adrift, but it doesn't matter. As soon as you can, take the initial image, and start working on it. Do not make efforts to try to remind yourself of what it means or what it is. Your mind works according to mental associations; let it work at its best without unnecessarily disturbing it: it knows what it must do. Manipulate the image, play with it a little. See if it looks brighter, or if it is smaller, or it is more pleasant. If it is a moving image, send it back and forth in slow motion or speed it up. When the initial idea always gets worse, replace it instantly with the second image.

Reorientation, also known as awakening, marks the end of self-hypnotic induction. Enjoy your new image, savor it as much as you like, and open your eyes when you have done this. If you have not given yourself any time limits before entering self-hypnosis, when you are satisfied with the work done, count quietly to yourself from one to ten, wake up, and open your eyes (Traversa, 2018).

The Benson Method

In his famous book, Relaxation Response, Herbert Benson describes the methods and results of some tests on a group of meditators dedicated to "transcendental meditation" to reach concentration (1975). Benson suggested a form of relaxation based on the mind's attention to a single idea incorporated in the Eastern disciplines. The technique includes the following steps:

- Meditate on one word, but you can choose an object or something else if you want to.

- Sit down in a quiet place and close your eyes. Relax the muscles and direct attention to the breath.

- Think silently about the object of meditation and continue to do so for 10-20 minutes. If you have lost the object of meditation, gather your focus again on the original thing.

- Once the set time is reached, open your eyes stretch yourself well for some additional minutes. To perform better, you will need to practice.

Benson proposes this exercise as a meditation practice. In reality, there are no differences between the hypnotic state and that achieved with meditation. It is one of the most straightforward self-hypnosis exercises you can do.

Here is another simple technique that the first hypnotists developed because it leads to a good trance in a reasonable time. It can be used to enter self-hypnosis in a short time.

- Begin to open and close your eyes by counting slowly. Open your eyes at the odd numbers close them at the even numbers. Continue counting very slowly and slowing down the numbering of exact numbers.

- After a few numbers, your eyes become tired, and you find it difficult to open them at odd numbers. Continue counting while you can open your eyes at the odd numbers. If you cannot do it, it means you are in a trance.

- Go deeper by slowly counting twenty other numbers. Let yourself go to the images, sensations, and words that come to mind. To wake up from the trance, count from one to five, and open your eyes at five (Stress Management Plus, n. d.).

These are examples of techniques, but no one is preventing you from devising others as long as the underlying assumption is maintained: concentration on a single idea.

Chapter 3   Hypnosis and Weight Loss

There are many benefits of conversational hypnosis, as the power of hypnosis will allow you to do many things you have never dreamed of. A hypnosis course will allow you to:

- manipulate everyone;
- follow your lead;
- get clients and customers to eat from your mouth;
- order respect;
- negotiate effectively;
- hold loyal lovers 24/7;
- make everyone consent to your point of view, including obedience from teens and kids.

There are ways to do it unconventionally, and if you know how to do hypnosis, you should do it. Everyone has the potential to hypnotize because it is usual among men and women, and they can do it easily if they complete a course on the subject rather than fishing in the dark. Using conversational hypnosis, as described by the name on the website, you can do things that others cannot conceive of.

By learning how to hypnotize somebody, you might be on the way to manipulating that specific person's power of hypnosis and making them follow the orders. A hypnosis guide will help you launch the exploration to read every customer like an open book. Only flit through the person's mind, and the entire person will be exposed to you like a journal.

You can understand and know the mind because you can learn how to interpret someone else's mind. With a single command, you can make people change, attitudes and, with a series of commands, you can gradually gain power over the individual and fine-tune responses to your wishes. You'll know what they think and how to turn a 'no' with a few commands into a 'yes.'

Hypnosis could allow you to do amazing things. You can quickly train people to respond to your voice tones the way you want and continually bid. You will know that you can fine-tune thoughts to strengthen relationships and build the missing bond between people. It's not a spell, but a course that's science, helping many people from coast to coast.

During daily interactions, you can use hypnosis because communication is how to manipulate people and offer. It will not only help you excel in your career but also help you load your day-to-day activities. Earlier, physicians were barred from hypnosis, but later, the rule changed and saved lives. You, too, will practice conversational hypnosis if you want to practice hypnosis and unlock the strength of your hypnosis.

The Power of Hypnosis for Weight Loss

Many people will try anything when it comes to weight loss-anything to stop regular diet and exercise. One of the more unorthodox approaches you do not find is weight loss hypnosis. Many hypnosis weight loss services claim to get rid of old habits, including overeating fast food. The way hypnosis works are to put you in a deep sleep where your mind is open to suggestion. For example, the hypnotist will convince you that you no longer have cravings or anything similar.

Some people believe that hypnosis is a crock, while others swear. Specific outcomes can differ if you were hypnotized successfully before; this form of hypnosis will work for you. When contemplating weight loss hypnosis, realism is critical. Hypnosis won't make you shed pounds overnight. Perhaps it will your cravings or make you want more exercise. The results will be sluggish.

One thing to stop when searching for weight loss hypnosis is hypnosis services in audiotape format. These programs say you can quickly get rid of your poor eating and exercise habits by listening to a tape repeatedly. If the whole thing sounds crazy to you, well, you're right. If you're seriously contemplating weight loss hypnosis, you can see a licensed clinical hypnotist and know whether it will function.

The nervous system is made up of your brain, your spinal column, and many interlocking nerves. The nervous system is super powerful and can critically influence your goal of burning body fat to determine which fuel is best for your body to use for its health and survival. Let's talk about two zones: the red zone and the green zone.

Red zone

The red zone is where we live stressed, busy, worried about the future; everything is urgent.

Green area

The green zone is ideal for relaxing so that our body works appropriately for digestion, repair, reproduction. As long as we focus on the green area, it will be easier for our bodies to lose weight.

How do you know if you are in the red zone? Here are some symptoms:

- You feel stressed most of the time.

- You have cravings for sugar or carbohydrates all the time.

- You don't usually sleep well at night.

- No matter how much exercise you do or how well you eat, you cannot burn body fat.

- You are tired most of the time.

- You feel that everything is urgent.

- You have digestive problems, and you swell quickly after eating.

- Your hormones are out of balance.

Being in this zone communicates to your body that you are not safe, in danger, and need to store body fat instead of burning it to survive. So, it is crucial to spend less time in this area to have better energy and decrease body fat.

Here I will tell you four solutions to correct the path and change to the green zone:

1.- Avoid caffeine.

Studies show that caffeine emits a signal to your nervous system that produces adrenaline. Adrenaline tells your body that it is in danger, in the red zone. Instead, go for some caffeine-free herbal tea.

2.- Analyze what the true urgency of things is.

I know there are emergencies like going to school for the children and the traffic is horrible but others like reading 100 e-mails. I assure you that of so many, only a few are important. Choose the important ones and read them calmly.

3.- Direct to the green zone.

Practicing Yoga, Taiichi, or my favorite, meditation/gratitude will take you directly to the green zone. When you are grateful, your nervous system cannot process stress and appreciation simultaneously, so it will block stress and automatically place you in the green zone.

4.- Be aware of your breathing.

Literal breath like a baby. Have you seen how they breathe when sleeping? When inhaling, expand your abdomen and then exhale slowly. This practice will communicate to all your cells that you are safe and that it is in this area where you will begin to use your body fat for energy. Try to do at least 20 of these breaths.

They are simple routines that you can start implementing in your day today. You will see that along with proper exercise (without stressing the body too much) and a diet based on excellent and whole foods, and you will begin to burn fat and have a very favorable change.

Chapter 4   How Effective Is Hypnosis for Weight Loss

Losing weight with hypnosis works just like any other change with hypnosis will. However, it is essential to understand the step-by-step process to know what to expect during your weight loss journey with the support of hypnosis exactly. In general, there are about seven steps that are involved with weight loss using hypnosis. The first step is when you decide to change; the second step involves your sessions; the third and fourth are your changed mindset and behaviors, the fifth step involves your regressions, the sixth is your management routines, and the seventh is your lasting change. To give you a better idea of what each of these parts of your journey looks like, let's explore them in greater detail below.

American women have a lot to think about besides losing weight, so a technique that interferes with your life as little as possible is the most practical approach to take. A practical approach like intermittent fasting also makes it more likely that you will continue to follow it through instead of quitting shortly after starting the way that many women do with diet and exercise. If you make exercise your primary technique for losing weight, you have to establish a new gym routine with relative frequency. Of course, all of us could find time in our schedules to do that, but the issue is that changing our plans so drastically makes us far less likely to keep on track with it. If the diet is your primary technique, you run into the same obstacle.

In your first step toward achieving weight loss with hypnosis, you have decided that you desire change and are willing to try hypnosis to change your approach to weight loss. At this point, you are aware of the fact that you want to lose weight, and you have been shown the possibility of losing weight through hypnosis. You may feel curious, open to trying something new, and a little bit skeptical as to whether or not this will work for you. You may also be feeling frustrated, overwhelmed, or even defeated by the lack of success you have seen using other weight loss methods, which may be what led you to seek out hypnosis in the first place. At this stage, the best thing you can do is practice keeping an open and curious mind, as this is how you can set yourself up for success when it comes to your actual hypnosis sessions.

Your sessions account for stage two of the process. Technically, you will move from stage two through to stage five several times over before you officially move into stage six. Your sessions are the stage where you engage in hypnosis, nothing more and nothing less. You need to maintain your open mind during your sessions and stay focused on how hypnosis can help you. If you are struggling to keep open-minded or are still skeptical about how this might work, you can consider switching from absolute confidence that it will help to have curiosity about how it might help instead.

Following your sessions, you are first going to experience a changed mindset. It is where you start to feel far more confident in your ability to lose weight and in your ability to keep the weight off. At first, your mindset may still be shadowed by doubt, but as you continue to use hypnosis and see your results, you realize that you can create success with hypnosis. As these pieces of evidence start to show up in your own life, you will find your hypnosis sessions becoming even more powerful and even more successful.

In addition to a changed mindset, you are going to start to see changed behaviors. They may be smaller at first, but you will find that they increase over time until they reach the point where your behaviors reflect precisely the lifestyle you aim to have. The best part about these changed behaviors is that they will not feel forced, nor will they feel like you have had to encourage yourself to get here: your changed mindset will make these changed behaviors incredibly easy for you to choose. As you continue working on your hypnosis and experiencing your changed mind, you will find that your behavioral changes grow more significant and more effortless every single time.

Following your hypnosis and your experiences with changed mindsets and behaviors, you will likely experience regression periods. Regression periods are characterized by periods where you begin to engage in your old attitude and behavior once again. It happens because you have experienced this old mindset and behavioral patterns so often that they continue to have deep roots in your subconscious mind. The more you uproot them and reinforce your new behaviors with consistent hypnosis sessions, the more success you will have in eliminating these old behaviors and replacing them entirely with new ones. Anytime you experience the beginning of a regression period, you should set aside some time to engage in a hypnosis session to help you shift your mindset back into the state you want and need it to be in.

Your management routines account for the sixth step, and they come into place after you have effectively experienced a significant and lasting change from your hypnosis practices. At this point, you are not going to need to schedule frequent hypnosis sessions because you are experiencing such substantial changes in your mindset. However, you may still want to do hypnosis sessions on a fairly consistent basis to ensure that your mindset remains changed and that you do not revert to old patterns. Sometimes, it can take up to 3-6 months or longer with these consistent management routine hypnosis sessions to maintain your changes and prevent you from experiencing a significant regression in your mindset and behavior.

The final step in your hypnosis journey will be the step where you come upon lasting changes. At this point, you are unlikely to need to schedule hypnosis sessions any longer. You should not need to rely on hypnosis at all to change your mindset because you have experienced such significant changes already, and you no longer find yourself regressing into old behaviors. With that being said, you may find that you need to have a hypnosis session to maintain your changes from time to time, particularly when an unexpected trigger may arise that may cause you to want to regress your behaviors. These unexpected changes can happen for years following your successful changes, so staying on top of them and relying on your healthy coping method of hypnosis is crucial as it will prevent you from experiencing a significant regression later in life.

Using Hypnosis to Encourage Healthy Eating and Discourage Unhealthy Eating

As you go through using hypnosis to support you with weight loss, there are a few ways that you are going to do so. One of the ways is to focus on weight loss itself. Another way, however, is to focus on topics surrounding weight loss. For example, you can use hypnosis to help you encourage yourself to eat healthy while also helping discourage yourself from unhealthy eating. Practical hypnosis sessions can satisfy your bust cravings for foods that will sabotage your success while also helping you feel more drawn to making choices that will help you effectively lose weight.

Many people will use hypnosis to change their cravings, improve their metabolism, and even help themselves acquire a taste for eating healthier foods. You may also use this to help encourage you to develop the motivation and energy to prepare more nutritious foods and eat them so that you are more likely to have these healthier options available for you. If cultivating the reason for preparing and eating healthy foods has been problematic for you, this hypnosis focus can be beneficial.

Using Hypnosis to Encourage Healthy Lifestyle Changes

In addition to helping you encourage yourself to eat healthier while discouraging yourself from eating unhealthy foods, you can also use hypnosis to help motivate you to make healthy lifestyle changes. It can support you with everything from exercising more frequently to picking up more active hobbies that support your wellbeing in general.

You may also use this to help you eliminate hobbies or experiences from your life that may encourage unhealthy dietary habits in the first place. For example, if you tend to binge when you are stressed out, you might use hypnosis to help you navigate stress more effectively so that you are less likely to binge when you are stressed out. If you tend to eat when you feel emotional or bored, you can use hypnosis to help you change those behaviors.

Hypnosis can be used to change virtually any area of your life that motivates you to eat unhealthily or otherwise neglect self-care to the point where you are sabotaging yourself from healthy weight loss. It truly is an incredibly versatile practice that you can rely on to help you with weight loss and help you create a healthier lifestyle in general. There are countless ways to improve the quality of your life with hypnosis, making it a beneficial practice for you to rely on.

The Benefits of Hypnotherapy for Weight Loss

It is hard to pinpoint the single best benefit of using hypnosis to engage in weight loss. Hypnosis is a natural, lasting, and profoundly impactful weight loss habit that you can use to change the way you approach weight loss entirely, and food in general, for the rest of your life.

With hypnosis, you are not ingesting anything that results in hypnosis working. Instead, you are simply listening to guided hypnosis meditations that help you transform the way your subconscious mind works. As you change the way your subconscious mind works, you will find yourself not even having cravings or unhealthy food urges in the first place. It means no more fighting against your desires, yo-yo dieting, "falling off the wagon," or experiencing any inner conflict around your eating patterns or weight loss exercises that are helping you lose weight. Instead, you will begin to have an entirely new mindset and perspective around weight loss that leads to you having more success in losing weight and keeping it off for good.

In addition to hypnosis itself being practical, you can also combine hypnosis with any other weight loss strategy you are using. Changed dietary behaviors, exercise routines, any medications you may be taking with the advisement of your medical practitioner, and any other weight loss practices you may be engaging in can all safely be done with hypnosis. By including hypnosis in your existing weight loss routines, you can improve your effectiveness and rapidly increase the success you experience in your weight loss patterns.

Finally, hypnosis can be beneficial for many things beyond weight loss. One of the side effects that you will likely notice once you start using hypnosis to help change your weight loss experience is that you also experience a boost in your confidence, self-esteem, and general feelings of positivity. Many people who use hypnosis regularly find themselves feeling more positive and in better spirits in general. It means that not only will you lose weight, but you will also feel incredible and will have a happy and cheerful mood as well.

Chapter 5   How Does Hypnosis for Weight Loss Work?

If you want to lose weight, you can rely on countless diets and exercise, but you can also rely on more innovative things in recent years. Let's take a look at a step-by-step guide that explains how to use hypnosis to lose weight.

Hypnosis therapy for weight loss can be used in a way that helps control hunger and nervous cravings, especially those caused by stress and the fact that you are eating at the same time. It is time to notice how this works, how many sessions should be done, and how it is ineffective.

Steps to lose weight using hypnosis

•   Hypnosis for weight loss is an effective treatment to reduce urges and desires and leave food vices, but the first thing to know is that it is `` help " and it can It is not a replacement.

•   Studies have shown that some people have lost more than twice their weight due to hypnosis. Not only that, they improved their eating habits and improved their body image. On the other hand, a meta-analysis conducted by British researchers found that hypnosis can help regulate the release of peptides that control hunger and satiety mechanisms.

•   Therefore, hypnosis is usually aimed at nervous, emotional people and those who eat at night. We often eat due to a lack of willpower and compensation (maybe we feel lonely, stressed, and depressed, food seems to give us temporary relief). The goal of hypnosis is to break this wrong link.

•   This treatment does not use a pendulum that swings in front of the nose to close the eyes. The patient and the hypnotherapist will have a conversation (about 25 minutes) during the hypnosis about the patient's goal, the trigger for hunger, and what diet will be followed.

- Also, experts suggest ways to deal with crisis moments when patients rely on food. Personalized therapist advice because there are different stories for each individual.

- However, rather than teaching that hypnosis has no desire, you need to know that you must understand that everything you want is not good or healthy to control your cravings.

- Once the therapy has started, most hypnotists offer about 12 meetings. However, you have to be careful because this probably doesn't seem right if you have not achieved anything after 3 or 4 sessions. Hypnosis is not always effective and does not work for everyone equally.

How Does Hypnosis Work

After a busy day in the office, everyone knows about chocolate, pizzas in a lousy mood: sweets, junk food, and the desire for certain foods to stroke your soul in stressful situations. It is not annoying at all-unless unhealthy eating is not a rule.

When a person comforts with a meal or wants to reward himself, this behavior pattern becomes so-called conditioning that quickly becomes a fixed habit. The body "listens" for unhealthy food and demands it in bad form of food desire and mood if it cannot be obtained fast enough.

This vicious circle leads to weight gain, frustration, and negative emotions polluting the body and mind. At this point, hypnosis begins.

Hypnotist treatment that breaks negative behavior and replaces it with new positive habits. This principle can be applied to fear of flying and nicotine addiction, and the desire for obesity and weight loss.

Instead of the desire for sweets and unhealthy eating habits, hypnosis was fixed in the brain behavior that supported the body while losing weight, for example, healthy eating and regular exercise units. Adverse side effects such as desire and the feeling of having to do without something should not have a therapy method, but rather hypnotize the natural senses for a healthy diet.

Everyone knows how it works. Adapting to life and the environment in modern society has simply "reprogrammed" our subconscious.

For whom is slimming with hypnosis suitable?

Regardless of the figure and physical condition, every person can go into the hands of a hypnotist to achieve his weight loss goal. However, hypnosis is beneficial in overweight individuals who have failed even after several attempts at classic diets - usually because they fall back into their old habits and eating patterns.

To effectively lose weight through hypnosis, you should also visit a reputable hypnotherapist you trust and can mentally engage in increasing your chances of success. Nobody can be hypnotized against his will. Those who, even unconsciously, resist hypnosis or the state of absolute relaxation cannot be treated and will not achieve satisfactory results in weight loss.

For all those who want to conclude with frustrating diets and consciously want to embark on a new weight-loss method, hypnosis is worth trying. Essential: Anyone who suffers from severe obesity should seek medical advice before starting hypnotherapy. Maybe several medical reasons such as hormonal imbalances or hypothyroidism. Even with morbid obesity, losing weight with hypnosis is not a suitable therapeutic approach.

How does a session go with the hypnotist?

During the hypnosis session, a therapist is responsible for putting the patient in a relaxed state, identifying the causes of the faulty eating behavior, and then manipulating it positively.

Reputable hypnotherapists recognize that they do not "show" their treatment and refrain from techniques such as lightning initiation, which puts the patient in a trance within a few seconds. Instead, the therapist tries to determine why the patient suffers from weight problems in a preliminary interview.

In addition to eating behavior, the focus is on the emotional and mental state - an essential prerequisite for ensuring a personalized hypnosis treatment tailored to the patient's needs. In the course of the preliminary discussion, the therapist determines, among other things, whether physical or mental hunger is the trigger for weight gain. Psychological hunger cannot be satisfied with food and is triggered by stress, grief, or frustration in many people.

The hypnosis itself then takes place either while sitting or lying down. Using a formula or concentration exercise, the hypnotist puts the patient into deep relaxation. The trance state between wakefulness and sleep is often described as a dream phase with full consciousness, in which the hypnotized, contrary clichés, but not will-less. On the contrary:

During hypnosis, the brain is particularly receptive - ideal conditions to replace old, unhealthy habits with new patterns of behavior, which bring the patient closer to his weight loss goal. The hypnotherapist guides the hypnotized with his voice through various everyday situations, revealing subconscious motivations for unhealthy eating habits and habits and anchoring new behaviors in his subconscious mind.

For example, in the trance state, the hypnotist gives you the message that doing sports is fun, and it's just part of life to go to the gym at least two or three times a week. Or that in the future, you will not feel like sweets anymore and only eat when you are starving. As a rule, the hypnosis session ends after around 30 to 90 minutes. Most patients report having a relaxed and pleasantly relaxed afterward.

Self-Hypnosis: What Do Hypnosis CDs and Co. Do?

Special hypnosis CDs or YouTube videos promise to achieve rapid customer success also from the comfort of your own home. However, such audio or video tutorials use common phrases like "I'm going to go without sweets" or "I only eat when I feel hungry."

According to experts, however, individual treatment is indispensable, especially in hypnosis, to lose weight. Indeed, some people are responding to the messages of self-hypnosis CDs. But if the weight problems have a cause other than excessive snacking, for example, self-therapy will be ineffective - and will at most make your wallet easier.

Studies confirming the positive effects of hypnosis in obesity always refer their results to meetings with a professionally trained therapist. On the other hand, it may be helpful to have the session with your hypnotist recorded and listen to the trance exercises at home (video, CD, or Mp3).

Can hypnotherapy help you lose weight?

Since there are only a few studies on weight loss and hypnosis, the effects of alternative therapy cannot be scientifically substantiated. However, some studies have proven the success of hypnotherapy for weight loss and as an alternative to dieting. As part of a study by the University of Tübingen, for example, 43 overweight women were given weight loss over six months. One-half of the subjects underwent behavioral therapy every two weeks, and the other received trance treatment and self-hypnosis guidance.

Although both groups were able to reduce their weight - the hypnotized women achieved significantly better results. Also, the study found that hypnotherapy had a positive effect not only on weight and body fat but also on overall health and greatly improved women's quality of life.

However, whether the pounds melt through hypnosis also depends on an inward willingness to engage in the unusual diet method: While many women believe that hypnosis is a complete humbug, Others notice a significant change in their eating behavior after treatment.

The testimonials of some patients even promise that hypnosis makes a weight loss of up to 14 kilos possible within five months and without the yo-yo effect.

Is hypnosis losing weight a natural alternative or an empty promise?

Whether hypnosis helps to lose weight permanently is not just in the hands of the hypnotist. At least as important as the qualification of the hypnosis therapist for customer success is the personal attitude of the patient.

If you are not in the mood for trendy diets and are open to embarking on an unusual therapy method, you may want to try it. Whether one achieves the desired weight with hypnosis, a sweat-inducing fitness program, or a long-term change in the diet remains - fortunately - alone the own decision.

Chapter 6   May hypnosis be more effective than diet?

Dieting only changes the food you eat for a while and limits your mindset. Thus, Meditation will help you tap into your inner feelings and respond to your craving with the ability to control yourself.

Not being on a diet also keeps your focus because you will be keen on what you eat and its benefits to your body. Meditation for weight loss changes the mind's perception, which triggers the inner self to respond to the choices and decisions. Dieting is restrictive and specific on the meals you are to eat.

It challenges the mind to believe that restriction in terms of food is the only path to weight loss. Meditation, however, is a healthy way of letting the reason be free to choose what is best, learn from mistakes, and focus on becoming better. It is possible to gain weight loss once one stops the diet process. It can offer both long-term and short-term weight loss needs. However, the disadvantage is you must know the calories to take per serving. If you do not see, you may take less, and your body will be deprived of the needed nutrient.

Tackling Barriers to Weight Loss

There are many barriers to weight loss, from personal to medical, support system, and emotional health. Meditation, if incorporated, will bring fruitful and healthy results. Dedication to overcome the challenges and to be focused on achieving your goals is significant. There are so many distractions, especially before you start your weight loss routine.

It takes discipline and resilience to manage a healthy loss program. We need to give weight loss the priority it deserves. Also, we need to realize the existence of the said barriers and their contribution toward our goal. The walls will determine our successes and failures.

Set realistic goals

When you set goals, ensure that they are attainable, specific, and realistic. It is effortless to work on realistic goals and achieve them for better results. However, if the plans are unrealistic, the success rate will be low since one will be discouraged. For instance, when starting with meditation, you can start with as little as five minutes a day and gradually increase it daily until you reach the maximum time, like sixty minutes.

The same applies to losing weight during the meditation process. You can start focusing on losing a few pounds each week and gradually increase until you reach your goal. However, as you set goals, realize that it is not your fault if they do not work out as you had planned, do your best and keep your focus.

Always be accountable

Once you have decided to commit to meditation to weight loss, don't shy away from sharing your plan with your support system and family. It ensures that the people you communicate with reinforce the commitment and form part of the support system. That way, they will feel part of the program and give support whenever there is a need. You can also use apps for reminders and timings; this way, you have a backup plan whenever you forget.

You can also use motivational bands whenever you achieve a milestone set. Being accountable makes you enjoy your successes, acknowledge your failure, and appreciate your support system. People thrive when they feel responsible for something, especially for something beneficial to their well-being.

Modify your mindset

Your thinking needs to be modified to be keen on the information you are telling yourself. Ensure that your mind is not filled with unproductive and negative thoughts, which will bring you down or discourage you. Do not be scared of challenging your ideas and appreciate your body image.

Your mindset determines your thinking and, in turn, creates a sense of appreciation or rejection. Our weight loss largely depends on our mindset. Do you believe you can do it? If you think you have all it takes, then absolutely nothing will prevent or stop you.

Manage stress regularly

Having a stress management technique should be part of one's daily routine. You need to develop a healthy stress-relieving mechanism that can help you live a stress-free life. Understand that meditation is a stress reliever in its own right as it helps calm the mind and soothes the body.

It can be used to manage stress and its benefits fully utilized to live a more productive life. Be able to handle stress efficiently. Pressure is not healthy for the mind.

If not handled, it can cause emotional problems and makes one irrational, moody, or violent. Be your own boss when managing your stress.

Be educated about weight loss

As you embark on meditation for weight loss, be educated about how it works; that way, weight loss will not be a struggle. You will be able to handle failed attempts as well as appreciate the progress made. You will know what you have been doing wrong and decide on the best meditation exercise for you.

Necessary: Misleading information may inhibit your general progress.

Weight loss need not be too expensive; neither requires a costly gym membership or enrolment in a costly meditation class. There are various self-practice meditation exercises that you can comfortably do at home. Different meal plans and diets may work for others though they may not offer long-term solutions or lasting behavior changes. Have the correct information that you need. Don't be misled by anyone posing that they are professionals in that field. Also, do not hesitate to do research online and compare notes. From there, you will be able to come back with something that works for you.

Surround yourself with a support system

Some people may be ready and willing to help whenever you want to start or even after beginning.

The support system may include your family, colleagues, friends, or social networks. These groups of amazing people may encourage and support you to meet your long-term goal. After you include them in your plan, they will feel accepted, offer opinions, and check on your progress. Analyze how things are going and encourage you to continue taking a little break when necessary.

Your support system should also include professionals in the field who will give sound advice and offer needed support and care. They will also help you discover the things hindering you and holding you behind and provide reliable information that can help you overcome. As you select the professional you want to work with, ensure they are easy to talk to and willing to participate in the routine you choose. You can also consider people who are ready to give an honest opinion as well as recommendations. Support systems sometimes have similar challenges that you may be going through at that particular time.

Their words of encouragement and best wishes usually would go a long way in motivating someone. Realize that ideologies may correspond with your point of view.

Chapter 7   Hypnotherapy for weight loss and techniques

Hypnosis is a great way to help those in need of weight loss. There are various reasons a person may be overweight. Some may range from behavioral issues or underlying conditions that will require to be addressed to lose weight successfully. Here, we will take you through a guide for a weight loss program through hypnosis and how to lose weight through meditation. After losing weight, a person needs to maintain it. We shall further discuss how hypnosis can help one maintain their new weight and avoid becoming overweight again.

Does Hypnosis Accelerate Your Weight Loss?

Those that have utilized entrancing to help in weight reduction have revealed incredible enhancements at the speed at which they had the option to shed the pounds. Here, we will talk about how this happens, utilizing suggestions from those that have attempted and succeeded.

Spellbinding is an instrument utilized by certain advisors to help individuals accomplish total unwinding. Specialists believe that the conscious and oblivious personality can concentrate and concentrate on verbal reiteration and mental imaging during a session. As an outcome, the psyche winds up open to recommendations and modifying conduct, emotions, and practices.

Since the 1700s, hypnotic treatments have been utilized to help people sliced from bed-wetting to nail-gnawing to smoking with anything. As we will research in this paper, Spellbinding examination has likewise demonstrated some guarantee to treat corpulence.

Mesmerizing might be progressively productive for people who need to get in shape than eating regimen and exercise alone. The idea is that to change practices like gorging, the psyche can be influenced. Be that as it may, it is yet being discussed how effective it tends to be.

What's in store from hypnotherapy

By clarifying how mesmerizing it functions, your specialist will most likely begin your session during the hypnotherapy. At that point, they will go past your personal goals. Your specialist can start talking in an unwinding, delicate tone from that point to help you unwind and make a suspicion that all is well and good.

When you have arrived at an increasingly open perspective, your advisor may propose techniques to help adjust eating or practicing rehearses or different strategies to accomplish your destinations of weight reduction.

With this point, certain words or the redundancy of specific sentences can help. Your specialist may likewise allow you to envision yourself by trading striking mental symbolism to accomplish targets.

Your advisor will help you escape trance and back to your beginning state to close the session. The term of the mesmerizing session and the full measure of sessions you may need will depend on your targets. In as few as one to three gatherings, a few people may see results.

Types of Hypnotherapy

Different sorts of hypnotherapy exist. For propensities, for example, smoking, nail-gnawing, and dietary issues, recommendation treatment are all the more as often as possible utilized.

With different meds, such as healthful guidance or CBT, your specialist may likewise utilize hypnotherapy.

Hypnotherapy expenses change depending on where you live and the specialist you pick. Think about calling forward to talk about choices for estimating or sliding scale.

Your protection business can cover somewhere in the range of 50 and 80% of affirmed experts ' treatment. Call for more data about your inclusion once more.

You can find authorized specialists by mentioning a referral from your essential doctor or via looking through the suppliers ' database of the American Society for Clinical Hypnosis.

Points of interest for Hypnotherapy

Studies demonstrate that a few people might be increasingly responsive and, in this way, bound to profit by the effects of entrancing. For example, an individual might be progressively inclined to be mesmerizing by certain character qualities, benevolence, and transparency.

Research has likewise found that mesmerizing helplessness ascends after age 40, and females are progressively open, paying little mind to age. Under the direction of an affirmed trance specialist, spellbinding is viewed as a protected practice with not many reactions, for example:

- headache

- dizziness

- drowsiness

- anxiety trouble

- fake memory creation

Individuals who are masters in visualizations or daydreams should converse with their primary care physician before exploring psychotherapy. Likewise, affected by drugs or liquor, the mental state ought not to be performed on a private person.

Extra weight reduction tips

- Here are a few things you can do at home to enable you to get more fit:

- Move your body on most days of the week. Attempt to get either 150 minutes of moderate action (for example, strolling, water heart stimulating exercise, cultivating) or 75 minutes of progressively lively workout (for example, running, swimming, climbing) each week.

- Keep a day-by-day dinner. Track the amount you eat, when you eat, and if you eat from yearning or not. Doing so can enable you to recognize evolving propensities, for example, fatigue eating.

- Eat vegetables and natural products. Go for five foods grown from the ground servings consistently. To check your craving, you ought to likewise add more fiber to your eating routine—between 25 to 30 grams every day.

- Drink water each day from six to eight glasses. Being hydrated, abstain from overeating.

- The inclination to skip suppers is safe. Eating throughout the day keeps up your digestion going incredible.

Chapter 8   The Power of guided meditation

As individuals, the first thing that we all crave in life is – peace. But peace is a broad term and one that leads to an endless list of questions. How do we define peace? What gives us peace? And most importantly, why do we crave it?

All of these questions are pertinent, and all of them have weight. You will begin to realize it is even more as you embark on your personal journey into the human mind in search of it. However, as you seek peace, it is crucial that you first try to understand how the human mind works and how meditation has multiple positive effects on the human mind, body, and soul.

While we think of mental health and mental development and automatically look to meditation as the perfect solution, it begs the question: Where did meditation come from? How long has it been around? Where did it originate? Interestingly, most of these questions lack a clear definitive answer even today, thousands of years since the practice was first adopted.

Some scholars have claimed that meditation, in some form or another, has existed from the beginning of humanity. However, India is an excellent place to start if you are looking for a more definitive answer. In this country, most commonly associated with meditation, Vendatism has been around since 1500 BC.

In China, Taoist meditation also dates back to the 5th and 6th centuries. Some scholars have dated meditation practices in the region as far back as 5,000 - 6,000 BC.

In the west, meditation didn't quite come about until the 1700s, though many Eastern philosophy texts. It wasn't until Swami Vivekananda, a Hindu monk, presented a speech at the Parliament of Religions in 1893 that this massive wave of interest in meditation brought us to where we are today.

Building Self-Awareness

For starters, let's focus on self-awareness. Take a minute and honestly ask yourself how aware your body reacts to specific situations. How do you respond to light? How do you react to fear? How do you respond to happy events? Take a minute and identify each of the previous physical manifestations of your mind and evaluate them – why do you respond in this way? Have you always acted in a specific manner? What has changed, if anything?

As you go through these questions in your mind, you may notice that other questions and thoughts will enter your mind that you didn't anticipate. It is actually very typical and natural. Even if you think that a specific view or trigger will cause your mind to think or work in a particular manner, in reality, it doesn't necessarily process the information in a specific way. It is why reverse psychology works on exact individuals and backfires on others – not all people react to the same form of stimulus in the same manner. Meditation allows you to practice introspection and truly identify how your mind reacts to precise triggers. It's almost as if your mind is doing a mental inventory of how you think, how you process, and most importantly, how you react.

Try to think of meditation as a form of mental yoga. The objective is to forge a more vital link between the mind and body. It ensures that your mind is more aware of how your body responds specifically to cues. Meditation helps us understand our sense of awareness. Helping ground us in the present moment allows us to act and think in a way that keeps us in the present.

Reducing Stress and Anxiety

It is just one benefit –meditation is not intended to enhance one's sense of self simply. In fact, a significant reason why so many people get involved in meditation is that they wish to use the practice to cure themselves of unwanted stress and anxiety that they might be dealing with.

Let's simplify this, shall we? Why do you think you are invested in meditation? What do you feel unsure or nervous about about starting your meditation program?

Try answering this instead – in the past week, what are five negative things that have impacted how you act, think, and react? Make a shortlist in a separate journal. Have you listed them for yourself? Good! Now ask yourself how often one of these thoughts has controlled your mind. Let's say you feel unhappy at work – how often have you thought of quitting? A lot?

How often do you think about how badly you want to change jobs? Almost always?

Most importantly, how often have you done something that would help you change your job or extract yourself from that toxic work environment? Odds are you just said never very quietly under your breath. Whether or not you feel ready to admit your thoughts to other people, you know exactly how often you sometimes obsess over the negatives in your life.

Do you ever wonder why you don't feel comfortable telling other people how often these negative thoughts come to mind? Think about it - if you don't like admitting how you are thinking, odds are that you already know, subconsciously or at some level, that what you are doing isn't good for you. Keep in mind that while negative things will continue to happen in your life, how far you allow that negativity to spread into your personal space is a decision you are constantly making. There is always a more productive way to deal with negative thoughts – if you feel you are stuck in a lousy job, instead of obsessing over the negative features of the job entails, train your mind to focus on the way out. Line up new job interviews consider talking to the human resources department or a supervisor; the point here is to actively do something instead of just letting things happen to you.

Taking control of the negativity surrounding you is vital to leading a healthier and happier life. This negativity breeds stress and causes anxiety to build in your mind. So, if you really want to live a stress-free, more nutritious, and most importantly, happier life, you are going to want to start by finding a way to reduce your stress levels and train your mind to focus on productive activities instead of anxiety triggers that you have built for yourself.

Honing Mental Clarity

Another common issue many individuals tend to deal with is – the lack of clarity that is predominant in today's world. For the most part, research has shown that multiple mental disciplines, such as yoga and meditation, can help control the mind and even improve it. Conditions like ADHD, a form of attention deficiency, have significantly improved with meditation and meditation-based activities.

While it is common knowledge that physical exercise can help keep the body in shape, people tend to forget that the brain needs the exact same thing. Neuro exercises or mental training activities can keep our brains in shape and weed out undesirable mental characteristics, such as depressive thoughts or anxiety.

One of the fundamental issues currently being studied by scientists is the subject of neuroplasticity. What is neuroplasticity, you may ask? Well, simply put, scientists have begun to discover that, contrary to popular opinion, an individual's brain is not shaped at the time of their birth – in contrast, the brain is actually constantly growing and learning, which is why it is possible actually to change our brains to specific forms of mental training. For example, one can retrain the brain to alter or improve multiple personality quirks, such as how attentive you are, how happy you are, how angry you are, etc.

Instead of considering emotions such as happiness, anger, or disappointment individual reactions, think of them as skills. You can train your mind so that you are more skilled at being happy or positive, although odds are you have subconsciously been training your mind to be the exact opposite. Neuroscientist Richard Davison of the University of Wisconsin conducted a three-month research program on the impacts of the Vipassana form of Buddhist meditation that deals with increased mental clarity and improving sensory awareness. On completion, he found that volunteers who had received Vipassana meditation as a form of mental training were much faster in their ability to identify and focus on detailed information. In contrast, individuals who had not participated in the training seemed less transparent and less stable in their ability to retain information. Meditation is now being seen as a form of mental exercise that helps individuals take advantage of the human brain's plasticity in a quantifiable and scientific manner.

Building Focus and Fortitude

However, it is not just mental clarity that is affected by meditation. In fact, a large part of meditation deals with building focus. While the science of the issue has clearly established that meditation can help enhance mental clarity by playing with the neural plasticity of the mind, it also does so on a more chemical level by releasing specific hormones to help counter your stress levels.

When you are stressed out, your body releases certain hormones to let your mind know overloaded. Once your mind starts to register that you are stressed out, the body releases adrenaline because it thinks your body needs more energy to help get you through these backlogged tasks. The only problem here is that adrenaline can work against you.

While theoretically, adrenaline should be helping you to get better and to do your tasks quicker and better. Adrenaline serves an essential function in our bodies, but unless we learn to control stress, adrenaline works against us. Instead of helping us get through stressful moments, excessive adrenaline increases anxiety and multiplies our stress reaction.

Chapter 9   Guided Meditation for Weight Loss

Meditation Exercise 1: Release of Bad Habits

Sit comfortably. Relax your muscles, close your eyes. Breathe in and breathe out. Do not cross your feet because this will lock you away from the desired experience. Hold your hands together to connect your logical brain hemisphere with your instinct.

Concentrate on your back now and notice how you feel in the bed or chair you are sitting in. Take a deep breath and let your stress leave your body. Now focus on your neck. Observe how your neck is joined to your shoulders. Lift your shoulders slowly. Breathe in slowly and release it. Feel how your shoulders loosen. Lift your shoulders again a little bit, then let them relax. Observe how your neck muscles are tensing and how much pressure it has. Breathe in and breathe out slowly. Release the tension in your neck and notice how the stress is leaving your body. Repeat the whole exercise from the beginning. Observe your back. Notice all the stress and let it go with a deep breath. Focus on your shoulders and neck again. Lift your shoulders and hold them for some moments, then rerelease your shoulders and let all the stress go away. Sense how the pressure is going away. Now, focus your attention on your back. Feel how comfortable it is. Focus on your whole body. While breathing in, let relaxation come, and while you are breathing out, let frustration leave your body. Notice how much you are relaxed.

Concentrate on your inner self. Breathe slowly in and release it. Calm your mind. Observe your thoughts. Don't go with them because you aim to observe them and not to be involved. It's time to let go of your overweight self that you are not feeling good about. It's like your body is wearing a more significant, heavier top at this point in your life. Imagine stepping out of it and laying it on an imaginary chair facing you. Now tell yourself to let go of these old, established eating and behavioral patterns. Imagine that all your old, fixed patterns and all the obstacles that prevent you from achieving your desired weight are exiting your body, soul, and spirit with each breath. Know that your soul is perfect as it is, and all you want is for everything that pulls away to leave. With every breath, let your old beliefs go, as you are creating more and more space for something new. After spending a few minutes with this, imagine that every time you breathe in, you are inhaling prana, the life energy of the universe, shining in gold. In this life force, you will find everything you need and desire: a healthy, muscular body, a self that loves itself in all circumstances, a hand that puts enough nutritious food on the table, a solid voice to say no to sabotaging your diet, a head that can say no to those who are trying to distract you from your ideas and goals. With each breath, you absorb these positive images and emotions.

Meditation Exercise 2: Forgiving Yourself

Sit comfortably. Do not cross your feet because this will lock you away from the desired experience. Hold your hands together to connect your logical brain hemisphere with your instinct. Relax your muscles, close your eyes.

Imagine a staircase in front of you! Descend it, counting down from ten to one.

You reached and found a door at the bottom of the stairs. Open the door. There is a meadow in front of us. Let's see if it has grass, if so if it has flowers, what color, whether there is a bush or tree, and describe what you see in the distance.

Find the path covered with white stones and start walking on it.

Feel the power of the Earth flowing through your soles, the breeze stroking your skin, the warmth of the sun radiating toward you. Feel the harmony of the elements and your state of well-being.

From the left side, you hear the rattle of the stream. Walk down to the shore. This water of life comes from the throne of God. Take it with your palms and drink three sips and notice how it tastes. If you want, you can wash in it. Keep walking. Feel the power of the Earth flowing through your soles, the breeze stroking your skin, the warmth of the sun radiating toward you. Feel the harmony of the elements and your state of wellbeing. In the distance, you see an ancient tree with many branches. It is the Tree of Life. Take a leaf from it, chew it, and note its taste. You continue walking along the white gravel path. Feel the power of the Earth flowing through your soles, the breeze stroking your skin, the warmth of the sun radiating toward you. Feel the harmony of the elements and your state of wellbeing.

You have arrived at the Lake of Conscience, no one in this lake sinks. Rest on the water and think that all the emotions and thoughts you no longer need (anger, fear, horror, hopelessness, pain, sorrow, anxiety, annoyance, self-blame, superiority, self-pity, and guilt) pass through your skin. You purify them with the magical power of water. And you see that the water around you is full of gray and black globules that are slowly recovering the turquoise-green color of the water. You again think of all the emotions and thoughts you no longer need (anger, fear, horror, hopelessness, pain, sorrow, anxiety, annoyance, self-blame, superiority, self-pity, guilt), and they pass through your skin. You purify them with the magical power of water. You see that the water around you is full of gray and black globules that are slowly obscuring the turquoise-green color of the water.

And once again: think of all the emotions and thoughts you no longer need (anger, fear, horror, hopelessness, pain, sorrow, anxiety, annoyance, self-blame, superiority, self-pity, guilt) as they pass through your skin, you purify them by the magical power of water. And you once again see that the water around you is full of gray and black globules that are slowly obscuring the turquoise-green color of the water.

You feel:

the power of the water:

the power of the Earth;

the breeze of your skin;

the radiance of the sun warming you;

the harmony of the elements;

the feeling of well-being.

You ask your magical horse to come for you. You love your horse; you pamper it and let it caress you too. You bounce on its back and head to God's Grad. In the air, you fly together, become one being. You have arrived. Ask your horse to wait.

You grow wings, and you fly toward the Trinity. You bow your head and apologize for all the sins you have committed against your body. You apologize for all the sins you have committed against your soul. You apologize for all the sins you committed against your spirit. You wait for the angels to give you the gifts that help you. If you can't see yourself receiving one, it means you don't need one yet. If you did, open it and look inside. Give thanks that you could be here. Get back on your horse and fly back to the meadow. Find the white gravel path and head back down to the door to your stairs. Look at the grass in the field. Notice if there are any flowers. If so, describe the colors, bush or tree, and whatever you see in the distance. Feel the power of the Earth flowing through your soles, the breeze stroking your skin, the warmth of the sun radiating toward you. Feel the harmony of the elements and your state of wellbeing. You arrive at the door, open it, and head up the stairs. Count from one to ten. You are back, move your fingers slowly, open your eyes.

Meditation Exercise 3: Weight Loss

Concentrate on your back now and notice how you feel in the bed or chair you are sitting in. Take a deep breath and let your stress leave your body. Now focus on your neck. Observe how your neck is joined to your shoulders. Lift your shoulders slowly. Breathe in slowly and release it. Feel how your shoulders loosen. Lift your shoulders again a little bit, then let them relax. Observe how your neck muscles are tensing and how much pressure it has. Breathe in and breathe out slowly. Release the tension in your neck and notice how the stress is leaving your body. Repeat the whole exercise from the beginning. Observe your back. Notice all the stress and let it go with a deep breath. Focus on your shoulders and neck again. Lift your shoulders and hold them for some moments, then rerelease your shoulders and let all the stress go away. Sense how the pressure is going away. Now, place your attention on your back. Feel how comfortable it is. Focus on your whole body. While breathing in, let relaxation come in, and while you are breathing out, let frustration leave your body. Notice how much you are relaxed.

Concentrate on your inner self. Breathe slowly and release it. Calm down your mind. Observe your thoughts. Don't go with them because you aim to observe them and not to be involved. It's time to let go of your overweight self that you are not feeling good about. Imagine yourself as you are now. See yourself in every detail. Describe your hair, the color of your clothes, your eyes. See your face, your nose, your mouth. Set aside this image for a moment. Now imagine yourself as you would like to be in the future. See yourself in every detail. Describe your hair, the color of your clothes, your eyes. See your face, your nose, your mouth. Imagine that your new self approaches your present self and pampers it. See that your unique self hugs your current self. Feel the love that is spread in the air. Now see that your present self leaves the scene, and your new self takes its place. See and feel how happy and satisfied you are. You believe that you can become this beautiful new self. You breathe in this image and place it in your soul. This image will always be with you and flow through your whole body. You want to be this new self. You can be this new self.

Chapter 10 50/100 positive affirmations for weight loss

Affirmations are necessary when you want to focus on another thought pattern. During claims, you phrase your statements positively, attach personal meaning to them, and repeat them to yourself multiple times throughout the day. Corresponding emotion helps the subconscious to understand the words and believe them as the new status quo. At first, getting your conscious mind on board with affirmations that may seem far-fetched can be difficult. As time goes on, however, the power of these affirmations has taken root in your subconscious, and you start to believe them to be true even with your rational mind.

You should change your lifestyle if you want to have experience permanent weight loss or control. Powerful affirmations are essential in helping to change your lifestyle slowly.

Thus, it would help if you practiced regular affirmations for weight loss to realize your dream of losing weight. Notably, weight control is a direct function of your lifestyle because you are solely responsible for your own behavior. In other words, your weight is determined by your mental attitude, rest and sleep, physical exertion, your manner, and frequency of eating.

You can use effective weight loss affirmations to be able to initiate these measures from your mind. Thus, you should change your thinking; otherwise, no form of dieting will ever help. Weight loss affirmations are significant in your mind, as they allow you to become a comfort in your desired weight.

It would be best if you also considered the words of your affirmations to ensure that you focus on the solution and not the problem. For instance, you shouldn't say "I am not that fat" because you're saying that is the problem. Instead, you should focus on the solution and say words such as "I am getting slimmer" or "I am losing weight every day."

Try to write down some healthy weight affirmations or take a cue from the samples in this book. You repeat these words repeatedly, which will help show that you are determined to take the bold step of living and fitter life.

So here are the words:

I weigh _______ pounds: this affirmation states the desired weight in your mind instantly, and as you repeat the words, you are reminding yourself about your destiny and all measures you should take.

I will achieve my ideal weight to enhance my physical fitness: you embrace a lighter weight and improve your physical activity.

I love eating healthy food because they help me to be able to attain my ideal weight: This statement promotes healthy eating and cravings for healthy food.

I ease digestion by chewing all my food to reach my ideal weight: This affirmation is perfect to say before every meal because it guides the rate and amount of food you consume.

I control my weight by combining healthy eating; it helps me manage my appetite and portion sizes. It is great to repeat this specific affirmation with others in front of a mirror to remind your subconscious mind about your goals. Also, these affirmations work best when you're meditating or in a trance state. The combination will help to do wonders in your weight loss endeavor.

Beliefs are formed by repetitive thought that has been nourished over and over for an extended period. Affirmations are positively charged proclamations or pronouncements repeated several through the day, every day. These words are often terse, straightforward, memorable, and repetitive. Affirmations are phrased in the present tense, and they lead to belief. The most crucial element of any self-improvement process is to set an intention. Muhammad Ali once said that "It is the repetition of affirmations that cause belief, and when the beliefs become deep convictions, that is when things start to happen."

Let's say you intend to shed some weight. That being the sole goal, it is paramount that all your efforts are focused on achieving it. Therefore, affirmative statements should be in the lines of, "Shedding pounds is as easy as packing them on," "I am what I eat," "A healthy mind is a healthy body," "I feel beautiful on the outside as I do on the inside," and so on. Keep in mind that not all the words you utter will yield results. For affirmations to work, they have to be coupled with visualization and a feeling of conviction. Therefore, it is advisable to focus more on positive thoughts than negative thoughts and for a prolonged period.

Remember to use words that resonate with you. The affirmations need not be empty for you. They ought to have a close relation and meaning attached to them. The formal statements for the appropriate situation go a long way in achieving success.

You can try repeating your affirmations before you go to bed. As the brain gets ready to go on "autopilot" mode, the subconscious mind becomes more active, thereby absorbing the last bits of information for the day. Repeating affirmations before you sleep makes you slip into dreamland in a more confident and relaxed state and helps to convince the mind.

You might begin to wonder why, if affirmations work, they are not used to get out of "tricky" situations. For example, if you are feeling sick, would you proceed to state, "I am cured. Am I well"? Affirmations work best with an aligned state of mind. If you believe to be well, it is more likely that you will begin to notice a decline in symptoms. If you do not believe in your affirmations, you will continue to battle through the temperature and other physical discomforts.

Finding the right words to use can be a stroll in the park; however, remembering to repeat these words severally could present itself as a challenge. The other obstacle you might face is having two conflicting thoughts. One of them is the carefully considered affirmation, while the other is a counterproductive negation. Try the best you can to disprove the negative thoughts but do not feed them time or energy. It will be quite challenging to believe affirmations, too, at the beginning. However, as time goes on, it will become easier to convince yourself. Practice makes perfect.

How Affirmations Affect the Mind

The act of repeating positive statements anchors your thoughts and energy, driving you toward their fulfillment. Affirmations program the subconscious mind, which in turn processes your reactions to circumstances. The more frequently you repeat the claims, become more attuned with your environment. You start seeing new opportunities, and your mind opens up to new ways of fulfilling your goals

Somewhere down in our unconscious minds, we've created solid thoughts regarding unfortunate practices. After some time, we may have prepared the psyche to accept that these painful practices are essential for keeping up our prosperity. Also, if the mind agrees that these practices are fundamental, long-term change is troublesome.

Stress or passionate eating is only one model. There are numerous affiliations that we build up that contrarily sway our relationship to nourishment. Some regular affiliations that forestall weight reduction include:

Nourishment is a solace cover; we use it to comfort ourselves amid stress or trouble. Eating occupies us from sentiments of concern, uneasiness, or anger. Indulging greasy, sugary, or unfortunate nourishments is related to festivities and other significant occasions.

Unfortunate or sugary nourishments are a prize. Indulging encourages you to pack the dread that you won't have the option to get in shape. Nourishment is a wellspring of amusement when exhausted.

At last, accomplishing long-term weight loss requires these main drivers to be surveyed, comprehended, and reframed. What's more, that is what hypnosis can enable us to accomplish.

50/100 Affirmations for Weight Loss

    1. I am fit, attractive, energetic, and healthy.

2. I am getting healthier, more energetic, and fitter every day.

3. I am stunning, inside out.

4. I care for myself by eating right, sleeping correctly, and exercising.

5. I take longer, more deep, calm, and relaxed breaths.

6. I love, care for, and nurture my body, and it cares back for me.

7. I am lovely, fit, and attractive.

8. I am completely relaxed and filled with serenity and peace of mind.

9. I am in a relaxed state of mind.

10. My body heals, replenishes, and repairs itself quickly.

11. I am beautiful in my body, mind, and spirit.

12. I go to bed early, sleep deeply, and am an early riser.

13. I create healing energy throughout my life.

14. I am healthy, relaxed, and happy.

15. I am healthy and confident and physically and emotionally strong and happy.

16. I am totally in control of my health, healing, and wellness.

17. I have abundant and inexhaustible energy.

18. I am capable of maintaining my perfect weight.

19. I am healthy in every aspect of existence.

20. I am a practical, healthy, fit, and energetic individual capable of handling anything that arises.

21. I will dedicate 15-20 minutes a day to exercise.

22. I feel vibrant, enthusiastic, and energetic every moment.

23. I enjoy eating nutritious, balanced, and healthy meals.

24. I have the complete power to control my fitness and health.

25. I love to eat healthy food and exercise.

26. I am the recipient of glowing health and a vibrant mind, body, and spirit.

27. I am thoroughly enjoying my daily exercise routine now.

28. I am fit, healthy, and active and practice regular exercises.

29. My body is fit and healthy, and all my organs function perfectly well.

30. Each day, I get closer and closer to my perfect weight.

31. I eat to fuel and nourish my body when required.

32. I have a strong heart and a formidable steel body. I am healthy, vigorous, energetic, and filled with vitality.

33. My body is a temple. It is holy, clean, and filled with a sense of goodness.

34. I am completely free from diabetes, high blood pressure, and any life-threatening disease.

35. I express my gratitude to God and everyone in my life.

36. I am healthy, wealthy, and wise. My body is healthy, my mind is brilliant, and I am always wealthy.

37. I eat healthy food that benefits my body.

38. I drink large quantities of water, which cleanses my body.

39. I feel good, my body feels good, and I radiate good feelings.

40. I have a healthy mind and a healthy body.

41. I have a strong heart and a healthy body. I am energetic and vigorous.

42. I treat my body as a temple. My body is clean, holy, and full of goodness.

43. My body is healthy, I am wealthy, and my mind is wise.

44. I surround myself with people who encourage me to be healthy.

45. I honor my body.

46. I am looking forward to a healthy old age because I take care of my body now.

47. I am grateful for my healthy body.

48. I enjoy living life.

49. I am worthy of good health.

50. I focus on positive progression.

Chapter 11 The Power of Affirmations

Positive affirmations are ground-breaking proclamations that we rehash to ourselves (either in our mind or so anyone can hear), and they are typically things that we need to occur. They are utilized to improve our internal reasoning and impact our conduct and the achievement we experience. Let's assume them usually with conviction and genuine conviction; your subliminal brain will, at that point, come to acknowledge them as natural. It will strengthen your new positive mental self-portrait and accuse you up of positive vitality. When your psyche begins to think something is valid, your disposition, conduct, and thinking will change to realize a perpetual change. Positive confirmations can be adjusted to any objective you wish to accomplish, including getting more fit.

Positive attestations are an extremely great device that you can use to assist you with shedding pounds. It very well may be trying under the most favorable circumstances when attempting to get more fit, particularly when you have melancholy or don't feel that great about yourself. Being overweight can cause a wide range of negative feelings that make it harder to remain spurred. Whatever you state to yourself significantly affects your circumstances and conditions. Truly the vast majority have no clue strictly how negative their idea designs are; have you ever gotten a brief look at your body in the mirror and felt your heart sink? Shouldn't something is said about when you state, 'I'm so fat and disturbing?'

These are both persistent instances of negative self-talk. Negative self-talk is a deadly inspiration critic just as being exceptionally terrible for your general confidence. Getting thinner takes persistence and duty, and if you need to succeed long haul, you deserve to take the necessary steps to remain positive and persuaded. So, what precisely are attestations? They are announcements composed or spoken in the current state that emphasize the result or objective you need to accomplish.

These weight reduction confirmations will assist you with moving your excursion towards getting in shape. I trust these 50 weight-reduction certifications proved to be valid. Make a point to bookmark this page for future reference.

When you have made your positive assertions, you have to put some time aside every day to rehearse them. There are many various ways you can do this. You may pick one articulation and state it for all to hear multiple times toward the beginning of the day and numerous times at night, or you should rehash it to yourself as you consider it for the day. As you recap your announcement, envision it is occurring: See yourself doing or feeling the quintessence of what your confirmation is stating. Make it as genuine as conceivable in your inner consciousness. As you picture and envision your objective, your intuition makes a psychological diagram.

Significant Affirmations for Weight Loss

At the point when you are prepared to accomplish your optimal weight, get more vitality day by day, and have higher confidence, this simple proficient recipe for creating weight reduction attestations is what you're chasing.

Stage One: Set Your Target Weight

Above all else, making compelling weight reduction certifications is deciding a clear objective load you would like to accomplish. Numerous individuals choose to get thinner essentially because they need to do only those get more fit. This point of view is that our psyches have been molded to consider losing anything as being awful. Consequently, when the intuitive mind knows about shedding pounds, it promptly relates weight reduction with a negative feeling, notwithstanding a negative perspective coming about because of sorrow issues.

Indeed, no one truly needs to get more fit, for they need to show up at their optimal weight, yet this is a direct, however critical differentiation when one needs to accomplish sharp weight reduction.

Stage Two: Decide What You're Going to Change

Positive weight reduction certifications or diet pills alone won't assist you with achieving brisk weight reduction. You should make changes in your eating routine and in your movement levels, which were, at that point, exacerbated by the downturn issues. Endeavors to discover an alternate route around this and accomplish brisk weight reduction will negatively affect that body that isn't justified, despite any potential benefits. Choose what modifications must be made to achieve you're objective other than picking the accurate weight. Doing this will give your intuitive psyche a specific arrangement of activities to actuate the body to take. It will likewise help with the downturn issues you are having as it provides the mind with something new to handle.

Stage Three: Build Your Affirmations

At last, form your confirmations after making sense of your objective weight and recognizing what transforms you should make to accomplish this. To do this, you should follow four fundamental standards:

- Make them in the current state

- Make them in the primary individual

- Make them agree (abstain from utilizing negatives like stop, won't quit, lose, not, no, and so forth.)

- Make them activity arranged

Activity arranged essentially implies that the affirmations address a specific action from stage two. As such:

"I'm eating increasingly regular foods and along these lines accomplishing my optimal load through reconditioning my digestion."

"I'm accomplishing my optimal load through a guarantee to opposition preparing and cardiovascular preparing."

"I appreciate expanded vitality and self-assurance in light of my pledge to appropriate sustenance and a functioning way of life."

See how these weight reduction certifications were completely composed utilizing the principal individual, agreed to articulations, activity arranged, and were in the current state. It is how you should keep in touch with them. At long last, you set these confirmations to work

Stage Four: Daily Rehearsal

Reconditioning the intuitive brain and reconditioning your body follows a similar arrangement of standards, and whenever followed, this will help with your downturn issues. For instance, if you chose to go to the exercise center a couple of times, you wouldn't anticipate accomplishing changeless outcomes. Hence, you need to invest in reliable action and adjust it into a piece of your way of life; furthermore, in particular, appreciate it, and you may even determine your downturn issues. When you have your weight reduction certifications made, state them resoundingly once every morning and night.

Chapter 12 How to practice every day

What's the key to taking out weight issues? I'll let you know. The mystery is to demolish the old subconscious squares, produce new idea designs, and fit your conscious and subconscious mind. Hypnosis can assist you in defeating the difficulties of subconscious courts.

You will feel all the more powerful. You will feel in charge. You will feel sure that you can control your weight with motivation and vitality to adhere to your weight-loss objectives. Hypnosis doesn't have any of the destructive or harmful symptoms of diet pills or surgery. If you pick proper eating and exercise plan and, at that point, reconstruct your mind with the goal that follows you're eating and movement program is not, at this point, hard yet simple, pleasant, and powerful, you will be fruitful.

Have a ton of fun practicing and eating solidly, with the goal that you quit causing self-actuated clash, stress, and demoralization. You will usually start doing the things that will bolster you in your objective to be sound and get in shape. It would be best if you disposed of the unfortunate idea designs that are making you overweight. These idea designs, which are put away in your subconscious mind, must be supplanted with solid contemplations and sound propensities so you will consequently do what you are required to manage while never mulling over it.

Does this sound confounding? It's, in reality, far less troublesome than you may figure. You will require about 10 to 20 minutes per day for a time of at any rate 21 days (the time it takes to build up a propensity).

Presently you can have the stuff to program your mind to shed pounds expediently. Hypnosis is one of the most misconstrued yet viable devices for self-change realistic on the planet today.

At the point when you state "hypnosis," a great many people consider Vegas enchantment shows or senseless stage acts. Those individuals in front of an audience were exceptionally picked for their defenselessness to the proposal. They would do nothing in front of an audience that they would not regularly do. They simply "don't mind" acting senseless in front of an audience for the consideration they get. If they don't perform, they realize they will be removed from the stage and back to their seat. Nothing could be further from reality. Hypnosis is essentially an exceptionally loosened-up perspective in which you are increasingly open to proposals. You ordinarily go into hypnosis commonly during the day.

If significant clinical affiliations have endorsed hypnosis to treat a disorder, envision how compelling it is to treat thought designs that hold up the traffic of the solid body you merit. The utilization of hypnosis to treat illness has been around for over 50 years. Indeed, the British Medical Association affirmed the utilization of hypnotherapy in 1955. The American Medical Association demonstrated its utilization in 1958.

In a 9-week investigation of three-weight the board gatherings (one utilizing hypnosis and one not using hypnosis), the hypnosis bunch kept on getting brings about the two-year development, while the non-hypnosis bunch demonstrated no different outcomes (Journal of Clinical Psychology, 1985). In an investigation of 60 ladies, the gatherings utilizing hypnosis lost a normal of 17 pounds; in contrast, the non-hypnosis bunch lost a normal of just .5 pounds (Journal of Consulting and Clinical Psychology, 1986).

Different examinations have demonstrated that including hypnosis expanded weight loss by a normal of 97% during treatment, and all the more critically, the viability expanded after treatment by over 146%. It has been demonstrated that hypnosis works surprisingly better after some time (Journal of Consulting and Clinical Psychology, 1996). Indeed, even Newsweek Magazine expressed, "The most effortless approach to get out from under negative behavior patterns is through hypnosis."

If you choose to utilize hypnosis sound tapes or CDs, study the content to decide whether the proposals bode well for you. Ensure there are no damaging proposals.

The mind doesn't hear "no or not," so the accentuation of the recommendation will be I WILL not eat stuffing nourishments. It will give you something contrary to your target. Continuously positively use suggestions. "I generally eat new nourishments that cause me to feel solid, fulfilled, and sound" is vastly improved.

It is critical to discover how you decipher the proposals. If somebody said, "That entryway ought to be shut," would you get up and close the entryway or simply think, no doubt it most likely ought to be shut and let another person close it. If you got up and shut the entrance, it implies you "surmised" that you should complete the entryway. A few people don't care to be determined what to do (direct proposals). You might be increasingly effective in making your sound. You could play a loosening up the sound and afterward peruse or work out your suggestions.

The best time for your mind to acknowledge these positive recommendations is in the first part of the day when getting up and in the night before hitting the sack. You need a tranquil space where you won't have to interfere. If you have a ton of movement in your home, you may need to discover a room where you can close the entryway and be undisturbed. It is for just 10 to 20 minutes.

For the vast majority, hypnosis is certifiably not a one-time fix. The impacts of hypnosis are aggregate. The more hypnosis is drilled with post-hypnotic proposals, the more changeless the outcomes become. Not very many individuals can be spellbound once and stop smoking or get thinner. If they do, they, as a rule, build up another propensity to supplant the one they simply halted. Numerous individuals who quit smoking begin to indulge. They just replaced one undesirable tendency with another. If you found the root(s) of the issue, there would be no compelling reason to substitute another propensity.

It may demonstrate significance to locate an expert prepared in hypnosis and the difficulties of weight loss. Working with an expert will assist you with comprehension and wipe out the prior programming.

To be compelling, particularly with weight loss, utilize the unwinding and self-hypnosis each morning and evening, changing and culminating your proposals as you get thinner. You might need to include different destinations after you show up at the weight you are OK with, alongside strengthening your good dieting and practicing propensities.

From the start, you should start with the complete unwinding; anyway, following a week or so, you will have the option to go into the casual modified state effectively by simply checking from 10 to 1. Continuously end your meeting with a proposal that you will feel better, better than anyone might have expected, loose and either alert, perceptive, invigorated, and brimming with vitality for mornings or open and ready to sleep if hitting the hay around evening time.

Ensure to have a paper and pen close by to record any bits of knowledge that ring a bell while tuning in or perusing your proposals. You may recollect things said to you as a kid that influences your conduct now. For me, I began recalling a ton of things that were said to me when I was a kid that I never thought annoyed me until I was particularly more seasoned. I simply didn't interface the things I recollected to my conduct. At the point when I remembered, I turned out to be furious. I understood the existence I missed by accepting what these individuals had said or letting me know as a kid and strengthened by others and occasions throughout the years.

Weight Loss Affirmations: Are They Enough and How to Practice Them

Weight loss affirmations would one say one is of the numerous everyday claims that individuals practice to develop themselves, yet would they say they are sufficient without anyone else to cause change, and how do you practice them successfully? This article examines what to incorporate with your positive affirmations for weight loss just as approaches to make them viable.

In the first place, when rehearsing weight loss affirmations or some other self-regard affirmations, recall that you are "working from the back to front." That implies that to roll out any improvement in your life, regardless of whether it is centered on your physical body or your funds, you need to change your mindset and internal mind (your subconscious) before any external switch appears.

While numerous individuals think about this idea, it's not constantly polished so that positive affirmations for weight loss or other self-regard affirmations function as well as possible. To "be slim," you must, as of now, "accept" that you are dainty, and this is the place the vast majority "tumble off the wagon" and quit doing their everyday affirmations when the external change doesn't come quick enough.

In this way, when you start, give yourself sufficient time to roll out the inward improvement with no "desire" to see any external change.

Next, you need to incorporate other everyday positive affirmations, for example, self-love affirmations, otherworldly affirmations, and affirmations of confidence and trust.

Chapter 13 The importance of Body Confidence

Self-love is probably the best thing you can accomplish for yourself. Being fascinated with yourself furnishes you with fearlessness, self-esteem and it will be by and considerable help you feel progressively positive. Likewise, you may find that it is simpler for you to experience passionate feelings once you have figured out how to cherish yourself first. If you can figure out how to adore yourself, you will be a lot more joyful and will figure out how to best deal with yourself, paying little respect to the circumstance you are in.

Self-Confidence

Self-confidence is just the demonstration of putting a standard in oneself. Self-confidence is a person's trust in their very own capacities, limits, and decisions, or conviction that the individual in question can effectively confront everyday difficulties and requests. Believing in yourself is one of the most significant ethics to develop to make your mind powerful. Fearlessness likewise realizes more bliss. Regularly, when you are sure about your capacities, you are more joyful because of your triumphs. When you are resting easy thinking about your abilities, the more stimulated and inspired you are to make a move and accomplish your objectives.

Meditation for Self-Confidence

Sit easily and close your eyes. Count from 1 to 5, concentrating on your breath as you breathe as it were of quiet and unwinding through your nose and breathe out totally through your mouth. Experience yourself as progressively loose and calm, prepared to extend your experience of certainty and prosperity right now. Proceeding to concentrate on your breath, breathing, one might say of quiet, unwinding, and breathing out totally.

If you see any strain or snugness in your body, inhale into that piece of your body, and as you breathe out, experience yourself as progressively loose, quieter. On the off chance that contemplations enter your psyche, notice them, and as you breathe out to let them go, proceed to concentrate on your breath, taking in a more profound feeling of quiet and unwinding and breathing out totally.

Keep concentrating on your breath as you enable yourself to completely loosen up your psyche and body, feeling a feeling of certainty and reestablishment filling your being. Experience yourself as loose, alert, and sure, entirely upheld by the seat underneath you. Permitting harmony, satisfaction, and certainty to full your being at this present minute as you currently open yourself to extending your experience of peace and happiness. And now, as you experience yourself as completely present at this time, gradually and quickly enable your eyes to open, feeling wide conscious, alert, better than anyone might have expected – completely present at this very moment.

Self-Love

Self-love is not just a condition of feeling better. It is a condition of gratefulness for oneself that develops from activities that help our physical, mental, and profound development. Self-love is dynamic; it develops through activities that create us. When we act in manners that grow self-love, we start to acknowledge our shortcomings much better, just as our strengths. Self-love is imperative to living great. It impacts who you pick for a mate, the picture you anticipate at work, and how you adapt to the issues throughout your life. There are such a significant number of methods for rehearsing self-love; it might be by taking a short outing, gifting yourself, beginning a diary, or anything that may come as "riches" for you.

Meditation for Self-Love

To start with, make yourself comfortable. Lie on your back with support under your knees. Put a cover behind your head, sit easily on a reinforce or a couple of collapsed bodies. For extra help, do not hesitate to sit against a divider or in a seat.

If you are resting, feel the association between the back of your body and the tangle. On the off chance you are situated, protract up through your spine, widen through your collarbones, and let your hands lay on your thighs.

When you are settled, close your eyes or mollify your look and tune into your breath. Notice your breath without attempting to transform it. What's more, see additionally on the off chance that you feel tense or loose, without trying to change that either.

Breathe in through your nose, and afterward breathe out through your mouth. Keep on taking deep, full breaths in through your nose and out through your mouth. As you inhale, become mindful of the condition of your body and the nature of your brain. Where is your body holding pressure? Do you feel shut off or shut down inwardly? Where is your brain? Is your brain calm or loaded up with fretfulness, antagonism, and uncertainty?

Give your breath a chance to turn out to be progressively smooth and easy and start to take in and out through your nose. Feel the progression of air moving into your lungs and, after that, pull out into the world. With each breathes out, envision you are discharging any negative considerations that might wait in your brain.

Keep on concentrating on your breath. On each breath in, think, "I am commendable," and on each breathe out, "I am sufficient." Let each breath in attract self-esteem, and each breathes out discharge what is never again serving you. Take a couple of minutes to inhale and discuss this mantra inside. Notice how you feel as you express these words to yourself.

On the off chance that your mind meanders anytime, realize that it is all right. It is the idea of the brain to curl. Essentially take your consideration back to the breath. Notice how your musings travel in complete disorder, regardless of whether positive or negative, and just enable them to pass on by like mists gliding in the sky.

Presently imagine yourself remaining before a mirror and investigating your very own eyes. What do you see? Agony and pity? Love and delight? Lack of bias? Despite what shows up in the meditation, let yourself know: "I adore you," "You are lovely," and "You are deserving of bliss." Know that what you find in the mirror at this time might be not the same as what you see whenever you look.

Envision since you could inhale into your heart and imagine love spilling out of your hands and into your heart. Allow this to love warm and saturate you from your heart focus, filling the remainder of your body. Feel a feeling of solace and quiet going up through your chest, into your neck and head, out your shoulders, arms, hands, and afterward down into your ribs, tummy, pelvis, legs, and feet. Enable a vibe of warmth to fill you from head to toe. Inhale here and realize that affection is constantly accessible for you when you need it.

When you are prepared, take a couple of more deep, careful breaths and delicately open your eyes after that. Sit for a couple of minutes to recognize the one-of-a-kind encounter you had during this meditation.

Chapter 14 What Happens During Hypnosis for Weight Loss

During hypnosis, your mind becomes open to any suggestions. Studies have shown that when in the hypnotic state, your brain is likely to experience exciting changes, which allows learning about the information you are receiving without thinking critically or consciously.

This situation leads you to detach yourself from your conscious mind, so stay focused and don't doubt it from what you are listening to. It is how hypnosis helps break down barriers that prevent you from shedding off weight.

In hypnotherapy, repetition is the key to success. It explains why many hypnotherapists provide you with self-hypnosis recordings, which you own to listen to repeatedly. The barriers in the brain are always powerful, and only through repeated hypnosis can you untangle yourself from the convictions. Hypnosis teaches the mind how to think differently about eating and food. The suggestions we learned can help you achieve the following:

Control Food Cravings

Weight loss hypnotic technique can help you to detach yourself from cravings and isolate yourself from unhealthy foods. For instance, during hypnosis, you might be asked to visualize how you will send away the desires. Suggestions can help in reframing cravings and teach you how to manage them effectively.

Success

Expectations of an individual dictate their reality. With the expectation of success, we are apt to take the steps necessary to attain success. Hypnosis can plant this seed of success in your mind, thus, giving you the unconscious power to keep yourself on course.

Positivity

Nobody likes negativity, and our brains are no different. Negative thoughts can spoil your ability and dedication to lose weight. Through hypnosis, you will become aware of the foods that you "can't eat." These foods do not help your body or health in any way. Thus, hypnotherapy will make you understand that you are not punishing yourself by abstaining from these foods, but you are doing that to improve your overall being.

Preparing for Relapse

Our minds have been trained to think that relapsing from a journey or goal is a sinful act, as it is a reason to give up. However, hypnosis gives us the chance of relapsing differently. The relapse becomes an opportunity to examine what went wrong, learn from it, and prepare for future temptation.

Modifying Behaviors

We can only achieve big goals by taking small steps at a time. Hypnosis empowers us to take action for these small changes, which eventually result in more significant goals. For instance, when you always reward yourself with high-calorie content and sugary foods, you will, over time, choose a healthier reward through hypnosis.

Visualizing Success

Hypnosis is considered a powerful motivator. It enables us to see results and explore how that impacts our emotional feelings. You might be able to visualize your future self telling others how easy it is to lose weight.

Getting Started with Weight Loss Hypnosis

•   Do you want to start your weight loss journey today? To begin, you have several different options. One of the options is to visit a certified hypnotherapist who will offer you face-to-face hypnosis sessions. Alternatively, you may schedule a session with a hypnotherapist via a virtual conference. Also, you may consider recorded hypnosis for self-training. The three standard hypnosis options include:

One-on-one hypnosis sessions— This session helps you identify the unconscious mental barriers that may hinder you from reaching your goal. Once you acknowledge your obstacles, you will be able to develop effective strategies to overcome them. Below are the things that happen during one-on-one hypnosis for weight loss: The hypnotherapist will guide you into reaching the state of hypnosis or deep relaxation. Once you feel fully relaxed, the therapist will be in a position to access your unconscious mind, including your survival mechanisms and innate instincts. The hypnotherapist will then use soothing words to explore your reasons for overeating and later suggest new thinking strategies through visualization. The process enables you to control any of the therapist's suggestions that you are not happy with.

•	Guided hypnosis sessions—This hypnosis technique entails hypnosis sessions that give you the advantage of mobility. You will start the sessions whenever you are ready and always use them on vacation or at home. The recorded sessions can take you through the process of weight loss, including suggestions that are valuable to you.

•	Self-conducted hypnosis sessions—An advantage of this option is that it is free of charge. In this case, you will take up the hypnotherapist's role by using a memorized script to induce hypnosis and, in the end, deliver positive suggestions. The main disadvantage of this approach is that it can be confusing at times since you may not be aware of what you are doing in the process; thus, you may not meet your weight loss goals.

What to Expect in a Hypnotherapy session?

Hypnotherapy sessions can vary in methodology and length depending on the practitioner. A session lasts 45/60 minutes, but patients with overweight problems need more time (3/4 hours). The general procedure entails lying down, relaxing with eyes closed, and letting the therapist guide you through suggestions, which can help you reach your goals.

A hypnotherapist can train your mind towards healthy food and away from unhealthy foods through the history of your weight loss journey.

Although you will be in an unconscious state of mind, the process does not make you do what you are unwilling to. Someone in a hypnotic trance will be between being asleep and wide awake. Thus, you are fully aware of the suggestions made by the hypnotherapist, and as such, can control or even stop the process.

Program Your Mind to Slim Your Body

Your mind holds the key to your life. You can either let your mind drive you to happiness or malcontent. The good news is that you have the power to reprogram your subconscious mind to lead the life you desire. When you were younger, your mind was a blank slate; it did not have any existing ideas, beliefs, or interpretation of events. Every time someone said something to you, the subconscious absorbed it and stored it away for reference. For example, if you were called fat, worthless, ugly, and embarrassing, all that negative information is stored away because the mind is always listening and impartial.

Now that you are older and know better, you believe it is merely a matter of getting rid of the false notions that your subconscious took hold of in your childhood and youth. It is easier said than done because the subconscious does not respond to the conscious mind. It is because your programming makes decisions for you. Take, for instance, you start a workout routine or a new diet. Your old programming reverts you to your old habits, and you fail miserably at your set goals. This habit can annoy and frustrate you, almost forcing you to abandon the quest for a healthier lifestyle. Before you embark on programming your mind to your slim body, keep in mind that you are already that person you intend to become. You need to develop the capacity to find them within yourself. To learn how to reprogram your mind successfully, you must:

Make A Decision

Decide on the exact outcome you wish for yourself. With clarity comes the power to shape your subconscious in the new paths to follow. Once you have settled on what you want for yourself, you offer your mental resources to fulfill your objectives. Please write it down.

Let's say you want to be 17-pounds lighter by summer, three months away. That is a clear-cut objective which you have set for yourself. Put it down clearly on paper and place it within sight to see it as often as possible. Therefore, when "external" forces try to sway you into indulging or binge eating, you remember that you have set a goal. You have decided to shed seventeen pounds in three months. All of your mental power is aligned to help you accomplish this task.

Commit

Once you have made a clear decision, commit to sticking by it. Commitment means allowing the decision to inform your choices. You may, however, expect to encounter fear. Fear is the biggest threat to success. The fear of failure drives people into giving up on their dreams-not loss itself.

Fear can lead to procrastination of your goals, which in turn feed the fear with negative thoughts such as, "I am better off not trying" or "Why should I risk disappointment in case I fail?" These thoughts cause you to feel even worse than you did before. The best solution for fear is facing it.

Failure is not the end of everything; it is a lesson in itself. Access the first trial, everything you did, and how you did it. Examine if there is a way to modify the exercise to alter the result. Therefore, fear should not hold you back from your goals. Your efforts should be coupled with a commitment to a healthier lifestyle, devotion to overcoming negative thoughts, and above all, commitment to yourself.

Modify Progress

Allow flexibility in your mental capacity. When you have committed to your decision, check the progress to see what works and can be amended. Striking a balance between alteration and overhaul can be difficult if you do not have a guide, a plan, or a mentor or sponsor.

Do not limit yourself to "It's my way or the highway" mentality. Having a peripheral vision can direct you to alternative possibilities and opportunities if problems arise during your course. Adjusting your programming to cater to these speedbumps builds your resilience to challenges. Your subconscious develops a winning attitude where failures become lessons, hurdles become catapults, and change is inevitable.

Reprogramming your mind to Overcome Limitations

To overcome limiting beliefs, you must first acknowledge them and accept them for what they are and their role in your life to this crucial point. It is of significant importance to get them because you cannot change what does not exist. Society repeats these beliefs, causing us to relate negatively with ourselves, food, money, etc.

When you realize that these beliefs do not define your worth, you will start to see your true potential and develop self-confidence in your abilities. You will feel free to win at everything in which you set your mind.

Chapter 15 Your Possible Weight Loss Block

What beliefs are holding onto your weight?

I am inferior

I am lacking

I am inconsequential, so I have to make myself big to be seen

Losing weight is too difficult

I will fail and put the weight all back on again

I must be so awful not to be able to control my eating

I want to punish myself

It is too hard to start dieting

My weight is ancestral, and I can't change that

My weight is genetic, and I can't change that

I am not good enough/I am not enough

I self-sabotage myself

I am worthless

I loathe myself

Healing negative beliefs

The best ways to heal negative beliefs and build confidence are the Emotional Freedom Technique (EFTTM) – Bach Flower Remedies Affirmations. Ask your guides and angels to help heal you. A pattern is a program that you have that is part of your personality. For example, in your character could be the thoughts:

I am not good enough

I am useless

I can't lose weight

I am not as good as other people

I am stupid

I am ugly

I am fat (remember, if you tell yourself you are overweight, you will be!)

I am to blame

It is my fault

I can't do anything right

I am a failure

It means that you block your weight loss as you feel that the task is too daunting, and you will fail. New patterns can be easily installed using EFTTM. A block is something that stops you from moving forward, and the biggest one of these is FEAR. The other one is being safe. If your subconscious feels that it is not safe, it WILL NOT LET YOU DO IT. So, if your subconscious thinks that losing weight is not secure, you WILL NOT LOSE WEIGHT! Also, if you feel you are worthless or do not deserve it, this will cause you to self-sabotage.

Healing negative patterns and blocks
The best ways to heal negative patterns and blocks are:

- Emotional Freedom Technique

- Bach Flower Remedies

- Affirmations

- Meditation

What is self-sabotage?

The term self-sabotage describes our often-unconscious ability to stop ourselves from being, doing, or having; being the person we want to be, doing what we want to experience or achieve, or having our goals and desires become a reality. Most of the time, we are unaware that we are self-sabotaging as it happens subconsciously. However, sometimes we are aware of that little voice in the back of our head that says, "you can't learn a language" or "don't be ridiculous; you can't lose weight."

Our subconscious mind is a powerful tool and always thinks that it is acting in our best interest. Stopping us from stepping into new territory, discouraging us from taking risks ensures that we don't get hurt, we are not humiliated, and we don't fail – that is why so many projects never get off the ground. Rather than playing to win, self-sabotage plays to avoid defeat.

The purpose of this aspect of the subconscious is self-protection and survival. It can even negatively affect your health if it protects you from more significant risks. Layers of excess weight have long been recognized as protection, and very often, the subconscious will use weight gain to protect you from perceived dangers you might be exposed to as a slimmer person.

For example, where someone has been abused as a child, the subconscious may add weight to make them unattractive (it thinks) so that the abuse is never repeated.

So, people may talk about self-sabotage about their weight because they eat emotionally and put on weight. However, sometimes self-sabotage will affect your hormones and organs, causing weight gain in people who eat only a modest amount. Sometimes people can lose weight but always put it back on just another method of self-sabotage. Once the perceived need to protect through self-sabotage has been healed and released, our illnesses and weight may disappear.

My experience of self-sabotage

I consulted a lady specializing in' muscle testing in my quest to lose the weight and water I had accumulated. When we asked, "Do I want to be slim" the clear reply was "no!" surprised me. So then started the journey of discovering why my subconscious didn't want me to be slim.

Why was I self-sabotaging?

During the long seventeen years in which I slowly cleared and healed the reasons for my self-sabotage:

- I had set up a self-punishment/self-destruct program because of what I had done in past lives

- I had set up a protection around me (weight and water) because of the sexual abuse, date rape, and male attention I had had – I didn't feel it was safe to be a woman

- I had several past life issues with starving to death and didn't want to die in this lifetime

- I had several past life issues with dying of thirst, hence the excess water in this lifetime to ensure that it didn't happen again

- I had a tremendous amount of other karma

- I thought that if I became a therapist, I could not trust myself not to hurt or experiment on patients, as I had hurt them before in past lives, so I was only going to be a therapist when I was 'slim.'

- I was frightened to take herbs as I had seen so many people die from them in past lives

- Because I had been persecuted in past lives for healing people, I thought I would be crushed in this life as well

- I was frightened of being powerful

- I was frightened to do the work I was supposed to do

- I was afraid that the book would fail

- Although I relate to my self-sabotage with weight and health, many other areas of my life are affected.

- I was always in debt and could never pay off my credit cards

- I never got the job I deserved and was very often out of work

- If I got a job, someone would always give me a tough time (karmic payback!)

When I had any treatments, such as red vein treatment or plastic surgery, it would always go wrong

Believe it or not, my subconscious created a reality where all of the above occurred – the subconscious is that strong. Even when I had released the attachments and got rid of my mother's influence, my subconscious was still following their examples, and as I strived to get better, my subconscious kicked in and made it worse.

So, my subconscious was negatively affecting all my organs and making them work so that I put on six stones and swelled up with water. My subconscious knew I could lose weight, and it decided this was the best plan of attack.

That's why some people lose weight and then put it back on. The subconscious doesn't always realize what is happening to begin with, hence the weight loss. It then kicks in big time in survival mode, and the weight goes back on. You would not lose six stone and then put it back on again – you might put back rock and then get it off. People blame diets or losing them too quickly, but it is simply your subconscious sabotaging you.

Emotional and comfort eating

When you read magazine articles, they always talk about emotional eating and weight gain. Some people do eat for emotional reasons and boredom. Some people do overeat, and there are explanations for this. You need to identify your emotional eating triggers and use a technique such as EFTtm to eliminate them. However, if you want to eat, wait for 10 minutes to breathe deeply, and you should find that the need to eat has gone after that.

However, I know a lot of slim people who overeat and drink too much. They fill for emotional reasons as well – slim people aren't perfect or without their own problems.

How often are you on holiday and you watch people eat an enormous breakfast, followed by a huge lunch and then three courses for dinner, plus booze, every day for two weeks? How often do you see a slim person eat a packet of biscuits or a bar of chocolate? ALL THE TIME!

You have to find why your subconscious doesn't want to lose weight and either release the reasons if these are past lives based or change your subconscious 'belief system' if they are more personality traits.

Removing the self-sabotage

When I was spending a considerable amount of money with therapists, and nothing worked, I did mention that I might be self-sabotaging myself. Most of them threw their hands up in horror and told me it was just an excuse to overeat (here we go again, I thought).

I read a lot about the Emotional Freedom Technique (EFTTM), and in the first paragraph, I read it mentioned self-sabotage. It was pretty amazing. However, my self-sabotage was so deeply ingrained that EFTTM just made everything worse as my subconscious tried to hold onto its control of me for a long time.

I, therefore, had to dig much more profound by clearing the attachments, past lives, and karma, and then I could use EFTTM and my other techniques to change my subconscious perception and its belief system that "I did not deserve."

Psychological reversal

I wanted to lose weight, but I didn't, and my subconscious was stopping me. You need to find out all the reasons why and release and heal them one by one. For this, you use the EFTTM psychological reversal techniques.

How are you self-sabotaging because my experience would lead me to believe that you are?

Habit of self-sabotage

I had a spiritual reading session and was told that the self-punishment had been healed but that I still had the 'habit' that needed to be healed and not recreated. I feel it is essential to include it in this book, as it would have never occurred to me that I still had the habit and could recreate it at any time. Our body and subconscious sabotage us so much that it becomes automatic and then a pattern. So even when the original stimuli are healed, the habit remains. So, remember to test whether there is a habit and then heal accordingly (usually the same way you healed the original pattern). Make sure you don't recreate the routine by repeating affirmations. If you feel yourself slipping back into 'deserving the pattern,' immediately cancel this feeling and ensure that you keep healing it.

Chapter 16 Comfort Eat

Eat Healthy and Sleep Better with Hypnosis

Make yourself comfortable.

Find the perfect sleep position.

Inhale through your nose and exhale through your mouth.

Again, inhale through your nose, and this time as you exhale, close your eyes.

Repeat this one more time and relax.

Sharpen your breathing focus.

Find stillness in every breath you take, relieve yourself from any tension, and relax.

Let your body relax, soften your heart, quiet your anxious mind, and open to whatever you experience without fighting.

Simply allow your thoughts and experiences to come and go without grasping at them.

Reduce any stress, anxiety, or negative emotions you might have, cool down become profoundly and comfortably relaxed.

That's fine.

And as you continue to relax, you can begin the process of reprogramming your mind for your weight loss success because, with the right mindset, you can think positively about what you want to achieve. It begins with changing your mindset and attitude because the key to losing weight all starts in mind.

One of the first things you must throw out the window (figuratively) before starting your weight loss journey is negativity. Negative thinking will lead you nowhere. It will only pull your moods down, which might trigger emotional eating. Thus, you'll eat more, adding up to that unwanted weight instead of losing it. Remember that you must break your old bad habits; one of them is negative self-talk. You need to change your negative mental views and turn them into positive ones. For example, after a few days of workout, instead of telling yourself that nothing is happening or changing, tell yourself that you have done a set of physical activities you have never imagined you could or will do. Make it a point to pat yourself on the back for every little progress you make every day; may it be five additional crunches from what you did yesterday. Understand and accept that this process is a complete transformation, a metamorphosis, if you will. This understanding is going to make the process smoother and less painful.

Aside from being positive, you should also be realistic. Don't expect an immediate change in your body. Keep in mind that losing weight is not an overnight thing. It is a long-term process and gradual progress. Set and focus on your goals to keep that negativity at bay. Losing weight needs consistent reminders and focus on proper mental preparations. Always keep yourself motivated. Train yourself to think good all the time.

Please don't compare yourself to others because it will not help you attain your weight goal. First and foremost, keep in mind that each one of us has different body types and compositions. There is a specific diet that may work on you, but not so much for the others. Possibly, some people might need more carbohydrates in their diet, while you might need to drop that and add more protein to your meals. Each one of us is unique. Therefore, your diet plan will indeed differ from the person next to you.

Comparing yourself to other people's progress is just a negative thought and will be unhelpful to you. Remember, always keep a positive outlook and commit to it before you start your diet. For the sake of your long-term success, leave the comparison trap. You're not exactly like the people you idolize, and they're not exactly like you, and that's perfectly fine. Accept that, embrace that and move on with your personal goals.

Be realistic in setting your goals. Think about small and easy-to-achieve goals that will guide you towards long-term healthy lifestyle changes. Your goals should be beneficial for your body. If you want to lose weight and keep it off indeed, it will be a slow uphill battle, with occasional dips and times you'll want to quit. If you expect progress too fast, you will eventually not reach your goals and become discouraged. Don't add extra obstacles for yourself; plan your goals carefully.

If possible, try to find someone who has similar goals as you and work on them together. Two is always better than one, and having someone who understands what you are undergoing can be such a relief! An added benefit of having a partner-in-crime (or several) is that you can always hold each other accountable. Accountability is one thing that is easy to start being lax after the first few weeks of a new weight loss program, especially if results aren't quite where you want them to be.

Write down a realistic timetable that you can follow. Start a journal about your daily exercises and meal plan. You can cross out things that you have done already or add new ones along the way. Plot your physical activities. Make time and mark your calendar with daily physical activities. Try to incorporate at least a 15-minute workout on your busy days.

When you become aware of a thought or belief that pins the blame for your extra weight on something outside yourself, if you can find examples of people who've overcome that exact cause, realize that it's decision time for you. Choose for yourself whether this is a thought you want to embrace and accept. Does this thought support you in living your best life? Does it move you toward your goals, or does it give you an excuse not to go after them?

If you determine your thought no longer serves you, you get to choose another idea instead. Instead of pointing to some external, all-powerful cause for being overweight, you can choose something different. Track your progress by writing down your step count or workouts daily to keep track of your progress.

Celebrate and embrace your results. Since the path to a healthy lifestyle is mostly hard work and discipline, try to reward yourself for every progress, even if it is small. Treat yourself for a day of pampering, travel to a place you have wanted to visit, go hiking, have a movie date with friends, or get a new pair of shoes. These kinds of rewards provide you with gratification and accomplishments that will make you keep going. Little things do count, and little things also deserve recognition. But keep in mind that your rewards should not compromise your diet plan.

You can also join an athletic event, a fun run, where you can meet new people who share the same ideals of a healthy lifestyle. You get to learn more about weight loss from others and also share your knowledge. You need to find a source of motivation and keep that source of inspiration fresh in your mind, so you don't forget why you embarked on this journey to begin with.

As you focus on your weight loss journey, keep your stress at bay because too much emphasis is harmful to the body in many ways, but it can also cause people to gain weight. When the body is under pressure, the body will automatically release many hormones, one of which is cortisol. When the body is under duress and stress, cortisol is released, it can ignite the metabolism for some time. However, if the body remains in stressful conditions, the hormone cortisol will continue to be removed and slow down the metabolism resulting in weight gain.

Everyone experiences stress; there is just no getting around that fact. However, minimizing stressors and learning how to manage the stress in your life will help you lose weight, making you a more attractive you! High pressure in anyone's life often brings out the worst in people. When you are trying to get a man, you want them to see the best of you, not the stressed-out you. While you are decreasing your stress level, you will want to increase the amount of sleep you get each night. Lack of sleep is a link to weight gain and because of this, ensuring adequate and appropriate rest is crucial when trying to lose weight. Sleep is vital for the body's general well-being and the ability for the mind to function, but it is also related to maintaining weight. If you are tired, make sure you sleep, rest or relax, so you are not prone to gaining weight. When a person gets more sleep, the hormone leptin will rise, and when this happens, the appetite decreases, which will also reduce body weight.

Gratitude is essential in this journey because it teaches you how to make peace with your body, no matter what shape, size, or weight it has at the moment. It makes you look at your body with complete acceptance and love, saying: "I'm grateful for my body the way it is." It stops you from beating yourself up for being overweight, unhealthy, or out of shape. Be grateful for this learning experience, accept yourself the way you are, and take massive action to regain your balance.

When you express gratitude, you vibrate on a higher energy level, you are optimistic and happy, and you are simply in a state of satisfaction. The more things you can find to be grateful for during your weight loss journey, the easier it will be to maintain a positive attitude and keep your motivation up.

It will also get you past those challenging moments when you feel demotivated to take action and stick to the exercising or eating plan.

It means that you start expressing gratitude for the aspects of your body you would like to have as if you already have them now. Be grateful for your sexy legs and slim waist. Be grateful for your increased energy levels and strength. Be grateful for the ability to wear smaller clothes. You get the drill. Feel the positive energy of gratitude flowing through your body as you imagine these things are true. By going through this exercise, you'll notice a positive change in your thought patterns.

With the personal growth you will achieve and the habits you will change in this hypnosis session, you will feel completely different. You will have more power, self–confidence, and love yourself more than you ever thought possible before. That's the change from the inside out. That's what lasts. And that's what truly matters.

Take a deep breath and allow your breath to return its natural rate as you return to your ordinary consciousness.

Chapter 17 Eating mindlessly

We eat mindlessly. The principal explanation behind our awkwardness with nourishment and eating is that we have overlooked how to be available as we eat. Careful eating is the act of developing a receptive familiarity with how the food we eat influences one's body, sentiments, brain, and all that is around us. The training improves our comprehension of what, how, amount to eat, and why we eat what we eat. When eating carefully, we are entirely present and relish each chomp - connecting every one of our faculties to value the nourishment. Past simple tastes, we see our food's appearance, sounds, scents, and surfaces, just as our mind's reaction to these perceptions.

The precepts of care apply to careful eating, too; however, the idea of mindful eating goes past the person. It likewise incorporates how what you eat influences the world. When we eat with this comprehension and understanding, appreciation and empathy will emerge inside us. Accordingly, careful eating is fundamental to guarantee nourishment supportability for who and what is to come, as we are persuaded to pick nourishments that are useful for our well-being and beneficial for our planet.

It is outstanding that most get-healthy plans do not work in the long haul. Around 85% of individuals with heftiness who shed pounds come back to or surpass their underlying load inside a couple of years. Binge eating, passionate eating, outside seating, and eating because of nourishment longings have been connected to weight put on, and weight recovers after effective weight reduction. Interminable presentation to stress may likewise assume a tremendous job in gorging and heftiness. By changing how you consider nourishment, the negative sentiments related to eating are supplanted with mindfulness, improved poise, and positive feelings. When undesirable eating practices are tended to, your odds of long-haul weight reduction achievement are expanded.

Steps to Mindful Eating

1. Watch your shopping list

Shopping mindfully – purchasing sound nourishments reasonably delivered and bundled – is a significant piece of the training. One thing you will probably find about careful eating is that entire nourishments are more dynamic and heavenly than you may have given them acknowledgment for.

2. Figure out how to Eat Slower

It is an intelligent thought to remind yourself and your family that eating is not a race. Setting aside the effort to relish and make the most of your nourishment is perhaps the most helpful thing you can do. You are bound to see when you are complete, you'll bite your food more and consequently digest it all the more effectively, and you'll likely end up seeing flavors you may find some way or another have missed.

3. Eat when Necessary

However, it might take some training to locate that sweet spot between being eager and greedy to the point that you need to breathe in a dinner. Additionally, tune in to your body and get familiar with the distinction between being physically eager and sincerely ravenous. On the off chance that you skip dinners, you might be so anxious to get anything in your stomach that your first need is filling the void as opposed to making the most of your nourishment.

4. Enjoy your Senses

The vast majority partner eating with simple taste, and many eat so carelessly that even the taste buds get quick work. Be that as it may, eating is a blessing to many faculties than simply taste. When cooking, serving, and eating your nourishment, be mindful of shading, surface, fragrance, and even the sounds various nourishments make as you set them up. As you bite your food, take a stab at distinguishing every one of the fixings, particularly seasonings. Eat with your fingers to give your feeling of touch some good times. By drawing in various faculties, the entire experience turns out to be significantly more completely fulfilling.

5. Keep off Distractions

Our day-by-day lives are brimming with interruptions, and it is normal for families to eat with the TV booming or one relative or another tinkering with their iPhone. Think about making family supper time, which should be eaten together, a hardware-free zone. It does not mean eating alone peacefully; careful eating can be an excellent mutual encounter. It just means: do not eat before the TV, while driving, at the PC, on your telephone, and so on. Consuming before the TV is a national hobby. However, simply consider how effectively it empowers careless eating.

6. Stop when you are Full

The issue with excellent nourishment is that it tends to be challenging to quit eating by its very nature. Eating gradually will enable you to feel full before overeating. Still, on the other hand, it is imperative to be mindful of segment size and tune in to your body for when it starts disclosing to you it has had enough. Gorging may feel great at the time; however, it is awkward a short time later and is commonly not beneficial for the body. With a bit of practice, you can locate the without flaw spot between eating enough, however not all that much.

Careful eating does not need to be an activity in super-human focus, but instead a straightforward promise to acknowledge, regarding, and, most importantly, get a charge out of the nourishment you eat each day. It very well may be drilled with a serving of mixed greens or frozen yogurt, doughnuts, or tofu, and you can present it at home or work. While the center turns out to be how you eat, not what you eat, you may discover your thoughts of what you need to eat moving significantly for the better as well.

Meditating to Heal Your Relationship with Food

The capacity to hold a broad scope of various feelings for the day is a test for many. We simply need to feel upbeat, yet the test is to locate that mystical parity of all we experience, decipher, and do. The most regular history of past weight reduction endeavors is ceaseless confinements, which require self-discipline and force. This perspective has a negative turn and does not draw out the best of us.

Meditation is a very accommodating device to mend enthusiastic eating. Meditation enables you to interface with your body. When you are in a condition of quiet and stillness, your state draws out the outer commotion of the world. Without these interruptions, it ends up more uncomplicated for you to drop into your body, construct, and support that association. When you have a solid association with your body, you are ready to accomplish things like unravel between physical yearning prompts versus enthusiastic appetite signals and perceive how to utilize nourishment for wellbeing and craving.

Stillness and predictable introduction to it enables you to construct your well of inward harmony and guidance. You will start to comprehend that you can exist outside of nourishment, weight, and everything in the middle. The more you reflect, the simpler you will discover it to drop into your body and associate with your higher self. You will be less inclined to go to binge eating as an approach to adapt to pressure and torment.

Meditation enables you to sharpen and use your breath. Breath resembles an inherent unwinding framework that you approach each moment of consistently. Breathing is the fastest method to accomplish a state change, which is the thing that your body is looking for when you voraciously consume food. Reflecting will condition you to depend on your breathing more on and then some, which means you will go after the shoddy nourishment less and less.

Please make this a standard practice; ensure you do it consistently first and foremost. Since at that point, the requirement for nourishment to fill this hole of the void will not be as large as you discover delight from other progressively self-engaging sources. Mindfulness will develop, and you will not just begin investigating yourself and your very own inward discussion. You will likewise expand your capacity to deal with the external mess. It accepts practice again with each new routine, but it can likewise mend your association with nourishment.

Chapter 18 Banning food

The entire intuitive eating approach revolves around listening to the body and keeping a finger on its pulse. If you cannot follow the signals your body is giving out properly, you will face problems implementing this lifestyle. Any dietician you go to initially or talk about intuitive eating will tell you that it's based on recognizing hunger and satisfying the needs accordingly. Earlier on, you read how there are different kinds of desire, and what you feel at times is not always what it seems like. Most of us are only familiar with physical hunger and spend our lives believing that it's the only type that exists.

The healthy living approach of intuitive eating has informed everyone that this is not the case. Your body experiences varying forms of hunger, and you do not always have to be satisfied with food consumption. One of the first core principles of this philosophy teaches people to honor their desire. It is about being aware of the biological urge which asks you to eat and then stop when you no longer feel empty. People say that this can get confusing at times as, during the initial stages, one is still trying to train their body and mind. If you think about it, exploring where and what kind of hunger may not be as difficult as one would assume.

There are no technicalities or complications which you have to unravel. Just consider these few points:

•When you feel hungry, wherein your body can handle the physical sensation? Are your stomach-wrenching and gnawing? If not, does your throat itch for something? Do you feel sluggish and tired? Sometimes, you might not experience anything but start feeling weak and experiencing a headache. If this happens out of nowhere, it's a sign that your body needs to be replenished with nutrients.

•Does hunger affect your mood or concentration? Do you find yourself thinking of food in the middle of work or a conversation? Those who have answered yes to both these questions, well, there you have it. When you feel hungry, your mood changes for the worse, your ability to concentrate on any task hinders, and if your thoughts are going out to meals and snacks, that is quite obvious.

•Are there any changes in your hunger when you travel, are stressed, or functioning on low sleep? To determine those, you need to closely monitor your body and try to remedy the source of the change because a disturbance in the eating pattern may be emotional hunger rather than physical.

An integral aspect here which people should be mindful of is that everyone experiences or feels hunger differently, and what one person goes through does not apply to the other. Remember that intuitive eating has no wrong answers, and it's a practice that brings about gradual progress, so if you do not get it instantly, there is nothing wrong with that because no one ever does.

On the other hand, hunger, which we talked about, is emotional and does not require any satisfaction, which comes from food. There are four types of desire that people generally experience; real, which you should immediately respond to according to the intuitive eating philosophy, and then emotional, practical, and taste.

In the beginning, you found out what physical and emotional hunger was about and how to successfully deal with each of them. Let's take this discussion a bit further. Physical hunger is perhaps the most important one here as it's your body reaching out to you and sending cues. It is also something that a lot of people fail to pay adequate attention to. You see, the diet mentality and culture have led to many treating their necessary hunger as an enemy. They consider it a challenge to overcome because otherwise, it would result in shame and guilt. Well, how can something so necessary for your survival be wrong for you? Hence, when your body begins to communicate with you, learn to listen.

The remaining three categories of hunger are, in a way, superficial. Emotional hunger is the trap that we have all ended up falling into. It consumes you in sudden, overwhelming bouts regardless of whether you have already eaten. The feeling is always there, and it makes itself prominent or visible when one goes through ups and downs in emotions. You look for comfort and security in specific, 'feel good' foods. As per the principle of intuitive eating, you have to figure out another way to honor your feelings without bringing food into the solution. When it comes to taste and practical hunger, there is an absolute divide of their validity. A few dieticians include distinguishing between hunger, while others tend to focus on physical and emotional.

Well, an extra bit of information does not harm, and it will only help you get to know your body in a better and more insightful way. Taste hunger is what you experience when you come across a food item or meal that looks good and tempts you to eat it. Take this, for example, you are at a restaurant and have already eaten a full meal, but then you see someone eating a colorful dessert, and suddenly you feel like eating it. You may not even be hungry anymore, but you are still going to end up consuming a portion of food because of its aesthetic appeal. It doesn't mean that you cannot eat it with intuitive eating; people do not have to question the value of their food items. They can eat what they want and when they want!

Practical hunger is something entirely different; in fact, you cannot refer to it as a feeling or state of being hungry. It's your mind telling you to eat before experiencing physical hunger. Yes, this is a real thing! Look at it this way, and sometimes, when traveling a long distance or having a long workday ahead, you end up eating meals even though you are not hungry. The mind anticipates your physical hunger and tells the body to fuel up before setting in, and the person ends up stranded in a situation where they cannot satisfy it. Snacking is an excellent way to deal with practical hunger, and light food items such as nuts, energy bars, or small sandwiches can help you contain your physical desire until you gain access to a full meal.

Intuitive eating is about validating and honoring hunger, which is how you make your way into healthy living and successfully get rid of any traces of diet culture.

The methodology dissects and analyzes hunger in great detail and implements for the best results. You have to concern yourself with it. Otherwise, it will just be another fad or trend similar to following a dietary plan. Intuitive eating is a philosophy that prides itself on standing up to dieting and telling people to live life as they want and according to a given set of rules by fitness gurus and instructors. One of the reasons why being hungry is given such importance is that it teaches people to live in the moment, enjoy the present and not run away from their cravings. As mentioned earlier, a sense of pleasure has to be derived, and it will only happen once you realize that your body requires it for optimum function. There are no rules that apply to foods you should eat or stay away from. Nothing is 'off-limits,' and you can indulge yourself without worrying about how the calories will add to your weight.

You see, this is where there is a stark contrast in the philosophy of intuitive eating and every other fitness plan. It doesn't consider the impact that consuming certain food items can have on you in the future. If you have tried any diet or fitness regimes, you know that they involve always keeping yourself in check so that you don't end up slipping and gaining weight in a few days. Now, this is not how the body's mechanism works, but it's what these diets have you believing. They engage people with the promise of a brighter future where they will be in excellent shape and looking good enough to feature on the cover of a health magazine.

This fallacy is what prevents people from living in the present and enjoying the little moments of life. You go to any party or celebratory occasion; the chances are that you will meet more than one person who won't be eating anything. They are probably not sitting down to try a delicious meal with others because they are thinking about the diet, getting to an impossible weight goal, or fitting into a dress they like. There is nothing wrong with trying to get in shape so that you can look good, but what most people do not realize is that in an attempt to accomplish something in the future, they miss out on what's in the present and within their reach. You are in a gathering, among people you like and great food, why not let yourself enjoy that rather than thinking about what will happen in a few months?

Intuitive eating allows flexibility, freedom of choice, and giving into cravings instead of waiting for them to go away. Now, you might think about how will you balance out a healthy lifestyle since you have acquired this approach? Well, it's pretty simple! Regardless of what it may initially sound like, intuitive eating restores the ecosystem within your body and makes you more aware than ever about your health.

Once you begin to ease into this approach, you will develop an eating pattern or habits around its principles and make beneficial physical activities integral to your day. You learned that intuitive eating perpetuates the idea of regular exercise and movement, so much so that you have to take some time out even during the busiest of days and carry out a simple activity. It could be something like walking around a block during lunch hour and stretching your body. The point here is not getting into shape but regulating the blood flow within your organization.

People, who are not inclined towards exercise and often become lazy when it comes to physical activities, will find that the intuitive eating philosophy makes it exponentially more comfortable to get started with them. It doesn't even matter whether you have exercised before in your life or not, and you can begin right from where you are! The methodology of intuitive eating is about putting your intuition into work and trusting your 'gut.' This is restricted to food and applies to physical exercise and movement.

Chapter 19 You don't exercise enough

That said, when you get going on a new exercise regimen, there are a few things you can keep in mind. These will help you get started and make sure you get the right kind of workout to suit your needs.

Firstly, the type of exercise you select will make a huge difference. To target your whole body, you need to pick out a wide range of workouts. Cardio is the first form, and you should spend three to four days a week getting some of this into your routine as it increases your heart rate and makes sure your heart gets some of the treatment it needs. Plus, the weight loss is really great because you can burn many calories in the process.

That doesn't mean certain forms of workouts aren't necessary. Weight lifting can also be done a couple of days a week because it also strengthens those muscles. Your metabolism will burn much faster during the day while doing everyday activities when the muscles are toned up. So, while you may not burn as many calories as you do with cardio during the actual workout part, weight lifting can be incredible for the metabolism benefits.

And on stretching, you can't forget. Take some time off your days, and do some stretching, like yoga or some other technique. It can help give the muscles a good time to relax after working so hard during the week, make them stronger and leaner and prevent injury.

Now, when it comes to how long you're supposed to work out, that will vary. When you want to lose weight, it's recommended you work out at least three days a week for 45 to 60 minutes. However, some people prefer to work out at whatever minutes for five or six days, so it's easier to fit into their schedule. When you are just beginning your fitness routine, and it's been a while since you've worked out, starting slowly is best. Ten minutes is better than nothing, and from there, you can build up. Never say you don't have time to work out; you can fit three or four ten-minute sessions into the day, and you've completed a full workout once you've done it.

Make sure the workouts you select have a lot of variety. Mix the stretching, cardio, and weight-lifting days together. Test out a host of different things, including some you've never done before. Mixing it up helps focus on various muscle groups that help with weight loss and make your workout easier to enjoy.

What if I don't have time to work out?

Some people worry they wouldn't have time to work out. They imagine spending hours at the gym to get the extra exercise you need to see the results you like. Yet you don't need to waste all this time in the gym with a successful weight loss program. You need to work out a few days a week and then find other ways to fit a little bit of exercise into your routine. Some of the easy ways you can add to your practice in more movement include: Get up every hour, rather than sitting at your desk all day long and never moving, consider getting up every hour for at least two to five minutes. Walk around the room, do some jumping jacks and run around just a bit. For five minutes of an eight-hour day every hour, you'll end up for forty-five minutes of exercise. You, too, should bring this around. Do some sit-ups and pushups during commercial breaks during your favorite show, and you will get an additional fifteen to twenty minutes each hour.

Park further away-if you need to take your vehicle, make sure you park far from the entrance. It might be just a few extra measures, but you do it a few times a day, and it really adds up.

Working out during your lunch-working out during your lunch break can be one of the best choices you can make. You can spend your lunch break just twenty minutes and then enjoy a nutritious meal for the rest. It won't take much time, so it can be an excellent way to stroll around the office or work in the local gym without adjusting your schedule too much.

Take the stairs — if you're working in an office just below the first floor, try going up the stairs instead of the elevator. Is the office is too far up to walk? Please start with a few flights and take the rest up the elevator. With time, you'll be able to increase your endurance and go up more flights of stairs.

Learn chair exercises – if you can't get up from your chair at work too often, learn a few basic practices that will help you work out your body without moving too often.

Add moves to chores—just cleaning the house can make you all sweaty. Make the movement intentional and add some things to it, and you're sure you'll get the additional exercise you want while making the house look fine.

Play at the park-take your kids to the park (walk there if you can) and then play at the park. Using the monkey bars, ride them, go down the slides, and more. You'll be shocked to see how much of a workout this will end up for you.

There's still time to add more exercise to your day; for that to happen, you just need to be a little creative. If you get up more often from your chair or sneak a few times during the day in the workouts, you're sure to get the results you want.

The Benefits of Working Out

There are plenty of perks you'll reap when it comes to working out. You'll see a massive difference in the way your body behaves and responds, you'll be able to lower your stress levels, and your attitude will begin to feel better in no time. Only ten minutes a day will make a significant difference in the overall way you feel. Some of the great benefits you'll be able to see when you start working out include:

Better mood: it's time to have a workout on those days when you're just mad at everyone and grumpy. Even if you feel down and down, it's time to get out there and enjoy a good workout. Ten to fifteen minutes is all you need to make your mood feel better, and if you can work out for longer, you'll find that your body feels so much happier and satisfied when it's over.

Clearer mind — there's just something to figure out that will clean the mind out and make you feel so much better. When you feel foggy or you simply can't get any more work done for the day, and it's only lunchtime, think about going out there and going into a good workout.

Healthier heart — your heart still wants some exercise. At least a few times a day, you want to use cardio to help the heart get up there and get stronger. Also, if you have to start slowly, you will find that working your soul with some good workouts like walking, running, swimming, and cycling will help you get that heart in shape.

Faster weight loss — you eat calories while you work out. So, the more calories you eat up, the quicker the weight loss becomes. Your metabolism should be more rapid, and it can eat up all the excess fat the remains in the body, so you'll be able to see some of those weight loss results quicker than ever before.

Toned muscles — sitting on the couch doesn't help your muscles be safe and robust. Instead, it makes them frail and fragile and wastes away. Neither do you just have to focus on weight lifting; stretching and cardio also have those muscles up and going, and you can see more strength in your body. Besides, these toned muscles will help speed up the metabolism, which is good whether or not you choose to lose weight.

Leaves you want more — beginning on an exercise plan may seem difficult at the beginning, and you may want to go out and do something else. You will learn to love it. If you can only keep up with the job for some time, you can see some fantastic results in the process. You'll start looking forward to the workout, for instance, to see how many results you can achieve. If you're someone who gets bored with the training, have a plan every few months or so to change it, and you're going to be perfect.

Although many people hate working out and putting all the time into it, there is a lot of good from daily exercise. Give it a chance together with the other parts of your Successful weight loss program plan to see how the outcomes improve.

Chapter 20 Self-Improvement through Self Hypnosis

Hypnosis is rewiring your brain to add or change your daily routine, starting from your basic instincts. It happens since while you are in a hypnotic state, you are more susceptible to suggestions by the person who put you in this state. In the case of self-hypnosis, the person who made you enter the trance of hypnotism is yourself. Thus, the only person who can give you suggestions that can change your attitude in this method is you and you alone.

Again, you must forget the misconception that hypnosis is like sleeping because it would be impossible to give autosuggestions to yourself if it is. Try to think about it like being in a very vivid daydream where you can control every aspect of the situation you are in. this gives you the ability to change anything that may bother and hinder you from achieving the best possible result. If you can pull it off properly, then the possibility of improving yourself after the constant practice of the method will be a few steps away.

Career

People say that motivation is the key to improving in your career. But no matter how you love your job, you must admit that there are aspects in your work that you really do not like doing. Even if it is a fact that you are good at the other tasks, there is that one duty that you dread. And every time you encounter this specific chore, you seem to be slowed down, thus lessening your productivity at work. It is where self-hypnosis comes into play.

The first thing you need to do is find that task you do not like. In some cases, there might be multiple, depending on your personality and how you feel about your job. Now, look at why you do not like that task and do simple research to simplify the job. You can then start conditioning yourself to use the simple method every time you do the job.

After you can condition your state of mind to do the task, each time you encounter it will become the trigger for your trance and thus giving you the ability to perform it better. You will not be able to tell the difference since you will not mind it at all. Your coworkers and superiors, though, will notice the change in your work style and your productivity.

Family

It is easy to improve in your career. But to improve your relationship with your family can be a little trickier. Yet, self-hypnosis can still reprogram you to interact with your family members better by modifying how you react to how they act. You will have the ability to adjust your way of thinking depending on the situation. It allows you to respond in the most positive way possible, no matter how dreadful the scenario may be.

If you are in a fight with your husband/wife, for example, the usual reaction is to flare up and face fire with fire. The problem with this approach is that it usually engulfs the entire relationship, eventually leading to separation. In this instance, being hypnotic can help you think clearly and change the impulse to say words without thinking through. Anger will still be there. Of course, that is the healthy way. But anger now under self-hypnosis can be channeled and stop being a raging inferno. You can turn it into a steady bonfire that can help you and your partner find common ground for whatever issue you face. The same applies in dealing with siblings or children. If you can condition your mind to think more rationally or to get into the perspective of others, then you can have better family/friends' relationships.

Health and Physical Activities

Losing weight can be the most common reason people use self-hypnosis in terms of health and physical activities. But this is just one part of it. Self-hypnosis can give you a lot more to improve this aspect of your life. It works the same way while working out.

Most people tend to give up their exercise program due to the exhaustion they think they can no longer take. But through self-hypnosis, you will be able to tell yourself that the fatigue is lessened, thus allowing you to finish the entire routine. Keep in mind, though, that your mind must never be conditioned to forget exhaustion; it must only not mind it until the end of the exercise. Ignoring it might lead you not to stop working out until your energy is depleted. It becomes counterproductive in this case.

Having a healthy diet can also be influenced by self-hypnosis. Conditioning your mind to avoid unhealthy food can be done. Thus, hypnosis will be triggered when you are tempted to eat a meal you are prepared to consider harmful. You're eating habits can change to benefit you to improve your overall health.

Mental, Emotional, and Spiritual Needs

Since self-hypnosis deals directly with how you think, it is no secret that it can significantly improve your mental, emotional and spiritual needs. A clear mind can give your brain the ability to have more rational thoughts. Rationality leads to better decision-making and easy absorption and retention of the information you need to improve your mental capacity. You must set your expectations, though; this does not work like magic that can turn you into a genius. The process takes time depending on how far you want to go, how much you want to achieve. Thus, the effects will only be limited by how much you can condition your mind.

In terms of emotional needs, self-hypnosis cannot make you feel differently in certain situations. But it can condition you to take in each scenario a little lighter and make you deal with them better. Others think that getting rid of emotion can be the best course of action if you genuinely rewire your brain. But they seem to forget that even though rational thinking is often influenced negatively by emotion, it is still necessary for you to decide on things based on the legal ethics and aesthetics of the real world. Self-hypnosis then can channel your emotion to work more positively in terms of decision making and dealing with emotional hurdles and problems.

On the other hand, the spiritual need is far easier to influence when doing self-hypnosis. Most people with spiritual beliefs can do self-hypnosis each time they practice what they believe in. For instance, deep prayer is a way to self-hypnotize yourself to enter the trance to feel closer to a Divine existence. Chanting and meditation have done by other religions also lead and have the same goal. Even the songs during a mass or praise and worship trigger self-hypnosis depending on whether the person allows them.

Still, the improvements can only be achieved if you condition yourself that you are ready to accept them. The willingness to put in an effort must also be there. Effortless hypnosis will only create the illusion that you are improving and thus will not give you the satisfaction of achieving your goal in reality.

How Hypnosis Can Help Resolve Childhood Issues

Another issue is that hypnosis can help with issues from our past. If you have had traumatic situations from your childhood days, you may have problems in all areas of your adult life. Unresolved issues from your past can lead to anxiety and depression in your later years. Childhood trauma is dangerous because it can alter many things in the brain, both psychologically and chemically.

The most vital thing to remember about trauma from your childhood is that given a harmless and caring environment in which the child's crucial needs for physical safety, importance, emotional security, and attention are met, the damage that trauma and abuse cause can be eased and relieved. Safe and dependable relationships are also a dynamic component in healing the effects of childhood trauma in adulthood and make an atmosphere in which the brain can safely start the process of recovery.

Pure Hypnoanalysis is the only most effective treatment method available in the world today for the resolution of phobias, anxiety, depression, fears, psychological and emotional problems/symptoms, and eating disorders. It is a highly advanced form of hypnoanalysis (referred to as analytical hypnotherapy or hypno-analysis). In its numerous forms, Hypnoanalysis is practiced worldwide; this method of hypnotherapy can completely resolve the foundation of anxieties in the unconscious mind, leaving the individual free of their symptoms for life.

There is a more profound realism active at all times around us and inside us. This reality commands that we must come to this world to find happiness, and every so often, our inner child stands in our way. It is by no means intentional; however, it desires to reconcile wounds from the past or address damaging philosophies which were troubling to us as children.

So to disengage the issues that upset us from earlier in our lives, we have to find a way to bond with our internal child. We then need to assist in rebuilding this part of us, which will help us be rid of all that has been hindering us from moving on.

Connecting with your inner child may seem like something that may be hard or impossible to do, especially since they may be a party that has long been buried. It is a relatively straightforward exercise to do and can even be done right now. You will need about 20 minutes to complete this exercise. Here's what you do: find a quiet spot where you won't be disturbed and find a picture of yourself as a child if you think it may help.

Breathe in and loosen your clothing if you have to. Inhale deeply into your abdomen and exhale, repeat until you feel yourself getting relaxed; you may close your eyes and focus on getting less tense. Feel your forehead and head relax, let your face become calm, and relax your shoulders. Allow your body to be limp and loose while you breathe slowly. Keep breathing slowly as you let all of your tension float away.

Now slowly count from 10-0 in your mind and think of a place from your childhood. The image doesn't have to be crystal clear right now but tries to focus on exactly how you remember it and keep that image in mind. Imagine yourself as a child and imagine observing younger you; think about your clothes, expression, hair, etc. In your mind, go and meet yourself, introduce yourself to yourself.

Chapter 21 Emotional Eating and Overeating

Emotional eating is something that we all do. Food is hardly ever unaffected whether we celebrate someone's birthday or mourn a loved one's death. Since we were young, comfort foods remind us that only the smell will make us feel comfortable and secure as it is a reminder of our childhood. When life is difficult or stressful, we still crave certain comfort foods most.

We don't know for most of us that we are emotional eaters or don't think it's that bad. For many of us, emotional eating does not lead to feeling inadequate or gaining weight. We can eat comfort for some of us and think it's not a big deal, but it is. For other people, emotional eating is out of balance and something that can dominate our everyday lives. It may sound like excessive cravings or hunger, but it's the feelings we experience that make us feel tired, helpless and add to our weight.

Comfort food gives us immediate pleasure, and our desire to taste it is stripped away. Digestion and sensation both take up a great deal of energy, and therefore, the body cannot do so. Comfort eating helps us not to face emotion because we flood our digestive tract with toxic waste.

Feeling a big empty hole inside us like we're hungry can be natural when we feel upset. Rather than discussing what that means – i.e., our feelings, we're stuffing it down. In culture, it seems we've grown afraid to feel so much so that we don't even know where most of the time, hiding from our emotions.

When we do not allow ourselves to feel like that, we must repress it. You can feel confused as you know and start allowing yourself to feel the feelings or emotions that come up and avoid stuffing down. It is because your body will release the past bottled-up feelings so that it will strike you hard. It is why it can be challenging to let go of emotional eating because, to move on and start learning to accept feelings for what they are, we have to get past the first initial "scare."

To be in the present moment is excellent and should be enjoyed to allow a feeling to wash over us. The more you allow yourself to be in the present moment and feel, the less you will be overwhelmed by emotions, and the less you will be afraid of them. The emotional strength would also decrease. You'll get mentally and physically stronger. When it is off your stomach, you'll feel so much better instead of replacing it with food.

Of course, it's not inherently easy to get to this level. Some people can split their emotional eating by properly nourishing their bodies to rid themselves of physical cravings and get help from others when they feel anxious or emotional – essentially substituting a human for the warmth instead of using food.

You need to be mindful of how and why you eat if you want to interrupt the emotional feeding. Take a day out to keep an eye on yourself, and what makes you hungry – eating from real hunger? Many people don't even get a feeling of real hunger!

When you catch yourself eating mentally, will you stop? Will you sit down and let the emotion wash over you instead of feeding – give yourself time to feel it and move past it? Or should you turn to someone to tell them how you think?

Don't get harsh on yourself. Emotional eating is typically something you've done from a very early age and is a part of your makeup. It is an acquired habit and how you learn to cope with the environment. It's going to take time to undo something so ingrained in you, but if you find yourself eating out of guilt – if you mess up – learn from it, don't feel guilty about it and move on. The first step is reconnaissance. When you know you're eating out of convenience, you can beat it up.

Journaling will also help you recognize you're eating habits. Write down the feeling before, during, and after a meal. What caused your hunger – was its actual starvation?

When you continue doing so, you should conquer the emotional eating within time and feel and care about yourself properly. If you find it too hard or overwhelming to combat yourself with emotional eating, you may try to see a counselor, or a great online program can help.

People eat for different reasons. To stop emotional eating, you have to know what it causes. Know what sensitive appetite causes circumstances, emotions, or locations. For the most part, emotional eating is caused by depressive thoughts and, at times, positive feelings, such as praising yourself for an accomplishment.

Food triggers mental.

Emotional eating is a big issue for many people who struggle with weight and typically shows an unhealthy relationship with food. Only if you understand what causes you to binge in this way will you break the pattern of emotional eating; you have to discover the circumstances and emotions that cause you to lose control of your eating habits. Eating for warmth to cheer up will turn into a vicious spiral as you could become more depressed as you pile up on weight, causing you to turn to food and make matters worse (and so it goes).

☐ Pressure – Once stressed, most people want to eat, and there's a good reason for that. When stress is chronic, it releases high levels of cortisol, a stress hormone. The cortisol gives you cravings for salty, sugary, and fatty foods — foods that will increase your levels of energy and pleasure.

Stress frees a hormone called cortisol, which can make us crave sweet or salty foods. Other hormones could leave us feeling an incredible desire for chocolate or carbohydrates. Although these cravings can be incredibly challenging to avoid, be mindful of the reasons behind your hormone-related needs. It can help you think about your choices and make better decisions until these feelings subside.

If you're an emotional eater, think carefully about your causes and what you can do to avoid them, and that will make a significant difference to your habits and wellbeing.

☐ Boredom – This happens when you're idle and have little to do about it. You should eat to get the hunger done. You're feeling hollow and unfulfilled to eat to combat hunger and get a sense of fulfillment.

☐ Childhood habits – Childhood memories of food can be recalled. Some parents use candy to reward kids for doing good things, and maybe your parents pay you with chocolate if you've got good grades. From infancy, you will pick up the habit.

☐ Social influences – Dinner with friends is a great way to socialize and have fun, but it can sometimes overheat. It's going to be easy for you to over-eat when your friends over-eat too, or you're going to overeat to calm your nerves. If you are motivated to eat by family members or friends, it is easy to do it.

☐ Filling emotions – Eating may be a way to suppress the negative feelings you can have, like wrath, guilt, depression, sorrow, etc. You get to lose those feelings by concentrating on food momentarily.

Control the Emotional Intake.

A straightforward method to perform this is to keep a food journal and a mood journal. Write down each time you know you've consumed unhealthy foods. Look back later on what feelings make you eat. You'll be able to recognize patterns or beliefs that make you overeat as time goes by. When you know what is causing your emotional eating, you will start avoiding it and finding ways to eat healthier.

1. Find other ways to fuel your emotions.

When you can't find another way to deal with your feelings without requiring food, so breaking this practice would be almost impossible. One of the reasons diets fail is that they give rational nutrition recommendations under the premise that lack of awareness is the only thing that stops you from eating properly. That form of suggestion only works if you can control your eating habits. It's not enough to recognize your causes and grasp your process to stop emotional eating — you need to find new ways to cope with your emotions. You can call or have a hangout with a friend who makes you feel better when you're depressed or lonely, visit places you like, read an interesting book, watch a comedy show or play with the cat.

2. When cravings arrive, pause.

It might not be as simple as it sounds because it is all you might think about when the desire for the food hits. You feel right there, and then, the need to feed. Taking at least five minutes before you give up on the craving gives you time to think about the wrong decision you're about to make. You can change your mind within that time and make a better choice. Start with 2 minutes if 5 minutes is a lot for you and increase the time as you get better.

3. Learn to embrace good feelings and negative ones.

Emotional eating comes from being unable to cope with the feelings in the brain. Find a friend or therapist who will speak to you about the problems and concerns you have. Being willing to accept negative and good emotions without having to include food would improve change.

4. Commit to healthy lifestyle habits.

Exercise, rest, and adequate sleep will make it easier for you to deal with any emotional or physical problem you may experience. Create time for at least five days a week for a 30-minute workout, relax, and sleep 7 to 8 hours a day. It's also essential to surround yourself with caring people who will empower you and help you cope with your issues.

The first thing to keep emotional eating in mind is the addictive effect food has on you. You may encounter cravings that often feel uncontrollable, and you may feel as though you are addicted to food much as a smoker is addicted to smoking. The trick is to properly control your emotions and feelings and train your brain not to respond to stressful or unpleasant feelings by merely eating food (your preferred brain drug) to calm down.

There are a few other practical methods and approaches that you can use to avoid emotional eating and lose weight, including: abandon the Diet!

Dieting ruins your metabolism, and you can eventually find yourself taking on weight. In reality, dieting will only work in the short run and will lower your fragile self-esteem.

Adjust your way of thinking.□

Chapter 22 Deal with your emotions without using food

First, abandon the idea that your emotional diet is terrible or uncontrollable. Not as much as most people do. Outside the context of food culture, we can even argue that dynamic food is not slandered as it is now. We go to the point where emotional meals are helpful.

An emotional diet is a way to let your body know something is wrong. It's pretty clever when you think about it. It's a clue, it's a way for your body to tell you something is happening, and you need to deal with it. It is a coping mechanism.

Food is closely related to emotions from a very young age. When the baby cry, parents provide them with milk. When you are a kid and win a dance contest, you go to celebrate pizza. There are cakes at birthday parties and weddings—ice cream when I broke up with my boyfriend.

When we are sad, funerals have sandwiches and sausage rolls. Using food to relieve unpleasant emotions is not inherently wrong. It's probably healthier than going home with a man who doesn't remember the name because of a blind drunk (don't say some of us weren't there!)

Importantly, drugs and alcohol Compared to misuse, gambling, self-harm, or sex addiction, food are very friendly. To not be embarrassed with these actions, we are all doing what we have to do (if you are suffering from these problems, ask for help you deserve what you need). The important thing is that food is a coping mechanism and an essential mechanism for that.

I'm concerned when food (or lack of food!) Is your only coping mechanism: if you don't know other ways to handle emotions, limit your dietary intake so that you can deal with it

A note on emotional overeating or restriction: The tendency may be unresponsive for many people when faced with challenging emotions. In many ways, this reaction is similar to eating to relieve negative emotions. Emotional overeating and overeating are both ends of the same spectrum.

The underlying reasons may be similar (unmet needs, lack of self-care), but they appear slightly different. In many cases, when people eat snacks in response to difficult emotions, it becomes a form of control. The world around them is messy, unfair, and unpredictable.

However, you can control what you eat and how much. Just as being overfull, the physical sensation of hunger can distract from more painful emotions and thus help deal with stress.

By building an emotional coping toolkit, nourishing the body is essential things we can do to show that we care about ourselves. On the other hand, withholding food can indicate a lack of self-esteem. You can recall how wonderful you are when you return to the list of 100 things you wrote about yourself.

Before that, let's consider what the emotional diet did to help you. I know it sounds strange. For most people, an emotional diet is a bad news, and it is something that you want to close quickly, if not immediately.

But here it is. If the emotional diet did not serve an essential purpose, would you have thrown it away? An emotional diet is not inherently wrong. It might have been the best way to deal with when something complicated happened in life. A maladaptive coping mechanism is just a representation of an unmet need.

If we can try and understand the purpose of emotional meals in your life, we get strong clues about your needs.

Think about when you use food to relieve unpleasant emotions or deal with difficult situations.

For example, you may have felt lonely, and food has helped distract you from loneliness or relieve that unpleasant feeling. Perhaps you are dealing with challenging things such as divorce, illness, bereavement, and you needed some sweetness in your life. Maybe you were angry at something, so you had to take it out with some food.

I know this may seem unnatural but go with it. In your diary, write all the functions of numbness, distraction, comfort, and food to relieve unpleasant emotions. Please write down your reflection along with it. Did this give you a clue about your own unmet needs? For example, if you are unfortunate, maybe the food

Emotional and Physical Hunger

Physical hunger: Now that I understand the signs and symptoms of physical famine, I will summarize it for the sake of safety.

- Build gradually

- Low energy

- Satisfied by eating something

- I'm hungry/irritated (I feel safe when I eat)

- Time has passed since the last meal or snack

There is also a taste of hunger. It is the feeling that you want to eat something just because you like the taste. It is usually met by having two Nutella or peanut butter spoons, some chips, a bowl of ice cream, some slices of cheese, etc. If you feel you need much more food to satisfy that desire, you may be seeing emotional hunger.

Emotional hunger:

- No physical hunger clues

- Particular craving

- I am not completely satisfied with the food (or I feel I need more food)

- It occurs immediately after the last meal or snack

- I'm looking at the refrigerator/kitchen

If you have confirmed that you are not 100% physically hungry, hungry, and not full of food, you may be experiencing emotional hunger. The tricky part is identifying what you are feeling. It can be not easy if you are used to stuffing instead of feeling, not feeling.

Ask yourself whether the feelings you are feeling are related to your eating desire. Here are some common emotional triggers that help food in that particular situation.

Abandonment-food is always there, and it is a reliable constant in your life

Anxiety – Use food to calm your nerves

Boredom – using food as excitement

Committee- "I deserve this because I had a ridiculous day."

Frightened-The food calms you down

Sky – food helps you fill the emptiness you feel

Inappropriate creating and preparing food can give you a sense of purpose

Joy – food is a celebration

Pride- "I got this snack because I received a promotion."

Loneliness-food reminds you of happy times with friends and even acts as friends

Sadness – peaceful food makes you happy in the short term – carbohydrates can boost serotonin

Reward – "I got this."

Emotion word wheel

It is difficult to recognize what you feel, especially if you are accustomed to using food to numb your emotions. There are two ways to try it according to your mood. The first is to use the circle of emotions in reverse to help put words or words into what you may be feeling. It might be easier to identify the feeling in the middle and narrow it down outward.

The feelings around the outside are a little more subtle.

If it's difficult to name your emotions, you can use the person outline below to identify where you feel in your body. Each emotion has a physical sensation. Like bodily conditions such as sleepiness and natural diet cues such as hunger and fullness, emotion is a component of cognitive receptivity.

The outline that feels emotion, maybe in multiple locations. Let's acquire a little creativity. You can give it a color, shape, or show strength by increasing or decreasing the emotion. You can print several outlines to map emotions over time and see if there is a pattern. You can also know whether there were extreme events, such as a fight with a partner.

UNDERSTANDING BODY SENSATIONS

Where emotions are in your body, there may be multiple emotions at the same time.

For each sense, consider the next dimension or characteristic of emotion.

Physical location: head, heart, chest, stomach, shoulder, neck, jaw, lungs, etc.

Shape: Circle, triangle, irregular blob, wavy line, spiral, zigzag, octagon, etc.

Color: This is entirely subjective. Choose a color that best reflects your emotions

Size: How strong emotions are felt may be reflected in the size

Once you have decided on the shape your feelings will take, draw it in a diagram.

Now you can see a visual representation of your emotions. Can you use a word from the word wheel to name it?

Can you identify the trigger of emotions?

Can you identify what purpose food serves to relieve that emotion?

Does this give you clues about what you need and how to meet your needs?

Chapter 23 Step to Avoid Emotional Eating

At some point, most of us engaged in emotional eating. Emotional eating happens if we eat to soothe wounded feelings or a stressful situation. Emotional eating can occur after a hard day at work, a fight with a loved one, or when the kids run around the house crying.

The first step to avoiding emotional eating is to know it is happening. Tell yourself many times during the day how you feel to alleviate pain. Recognize uncomfortable emotions or tension.

Find a way to transmit the feelings efficiently. Holding negative or detrimental emotions may lead to a later binge. Stopping during the day to determine your feelings can also help you quit unhealthy foods.

Second, prevent causes.

Think back to the last emotional eating moment. What happened just before you'd eat? Remember not being hungry and eating anyway? Should you still eat after a problematic job meeting or argument with a co-worker? Identifying and preventing emotional-eating activities can help reduce potential incidents.

Second, try doing something else when eating happens. By monitoring your emotional state during the day, you will be conscious of when emotional eating will occur and seek solutions. If eating fattening foods makes you feel confident and relaxed, build a list of other habits contributing to the same feelings.

Exercise is a meaningful way to promote positive feelings. Other suggestions like hot baths, reading a good book or watching your favorite movie. Place the activity list on your refrigerator to remind you of possible tips should a weakness occur. Journaling is another way to avoid emotional eating.

Tracking prolonged all-day feelings as anxieties, fears, and emotions will help you recognize causes. While keeping a list for a few days, look back for specific feelings that made you eat emotionally.

Another way to prevent emotional eating is to cut your servings in half.

If you've had a busy day and have a meal, place half-sized portions on your plate and assess how you feel after you've eaten. If you're still hungry, you might eat more, but if you're feeling depressed and looking for warmth, take a moment to consider your motives.

Assessing your appetite and emotional state will avoid over-eating. Remove comforts like white bread and processed sugars. Such foods mask unpleasant emotions and cannot satisfy you until the meal is finished. Need to drink plenty of water during your meal. Recognize when you're complete and stop.

Eventually, if you feed mentally, forgive yourself. When you keep thinking negatively about yourself, you're just inviting more tension and the opportunity to eat emotionally.

Weak eating habits take years to develop and are uncorrectable overnight. Act towards small goals and enjoy something other than food when you celebrate.

When I think of comfort food, it produces lovely delicious pictures of mac n' cheese, lasagna, chocolate cake, and ice cream sodas. Many people also turn to these homey childhood memories when they crave a familiar taste during a difficult or stressful period.

Food can be closely linked to feelings, but this connection is unhealthy for others. It's known as emotional eating, leading to weight gain, unhealthy food relationships, and even eating disorders.

Emotional eating is when a person turns to food to soothe or escape unpleasant feelings such as loneliness, tension, boredom, and sadness. Experts claim that 75% of overeating might have an emotional aspect. At the same time, most of my patients used food to change their moods; eating ice cream when watching TV alone or grabbing a candy bar after a frustrating workshop is understandable.

Most people don't even know they're pick-me-up stuff. Nevertheless, if this form of eating is standard, you may be setting up for unhealthy effects like weight gain.

Think about the last time you turned to your favorite food. Are you hungry? If not, your feelings-controlled actions. Emotional eating appears to induce feelings of remorse or regret, leading to more consumption.

Meeting true hunger doesn't make you feel bad. Emotional eaters often prefer to eat until feeling full. When you're hungry, you're possibly pleased with a range of foods. Many emotional eaters unexpectedly find themselves craving things like chocolate, cookies, salty chips and will not be happy until they eat them.

Most people go for years before realizing emotional eating's dangerous trend. They also pursue several weight loss programs without success because all the world's diets won't sever an emotional bond to food. If this sounds like you, be told you can change your actions and stop gaining weight.

The best way to avoid emotional eating is to acknowledge real hunger. Most people fear hunger, but stomach rumbling is not the world's end. You're unlikely to die of starvation if you let yourself go.

Consider this: eat until you're bloated until you're about three-quarters full. You should be content but relaxed. Then don't feed again until you feel hungry (generally, 4-5 hours). This exercise lets you understand your own hunger feeling. Emotional eaters prefer to eat so much they can't recall how hunger feels.

To get to the heart of emotional eating, keep a two-week diet diary. Not only do you record every bite you put in your mouth but find out why you eat and how you feel before and after.

For example, "I ate a turkey sandwich on whole-wheat bread because it was my lunch break and I felt hungry. I felt half full afterward, so I ate an apple and felt relaxed and happy." When things don't go so well, it's best to write it in your food log.

For example, "I ate a Snickers bar at 3:30. I was still full of lunch, but I was anxious because tomorrow's sales report is due, and I have to work late."

Look back after two weeks and notice some trends. Maybe you like to eat sweets in the afternoon as all workday tension starts to build up. You can find you're most insecure late at night after the kids go to bed. If you know the emotional eating issues, you can formulate strategies to make them more manageable.

If emotional eating gains weight, don't be too hard on yourself. Tackle the unpleasant feelings and circumstances when you first switch to food. Holding the food log and listening to the hunger signals was a great help to my patients battling this problem.

By making hunger-based food decisions, not feelings, you are likely to lose weight naturally. It would lead to daily healthy eating choices. Remember to recover from emotional eating and hit a healthy, happy weight.

Weight Loss Tips to Stop Emotional Eating

Emotional eating can hinder weight-loss efforts. But the good news is that you can monitor your eating habits and keep track of your weight loss goals.

Our most intense food needs also arise while emotionally weak. When faced with complex issues, tension, or just looking to keep busy, we prefer to look for warmth. But it's wrong to constantly use food to solve problems that we need to address from an emotional perspective, while food can give us temporary gratification.

Most emotional eating leads to binge eating, obese, high-calorie sweet foods that quickly lead to weight gain. Since emotional eating means eating to conceal or soothe unpleasant feelings, we are most at risk in moments of sorrow, boredom, anxiety, stress, and rage.

Emotional eating triggers: Major life events and day-to-day stress can cause negative feelings that result in emotional eating and throw off balance weight loss program. These causes may include, but are not limited to, sickness, income loss, family problems, relationship issues, financial distress, loved one's loss, and work-related stress.

We prefer to succumb to impulsive eating in moments of high feelings-grabbing everything we can lay our hands-on, whether we like it or not. In severe cases, our feelings can become so tied to the eating patterns that we reach for any available sweet food while anxious, without even thinking about it. If you're concerned about an occurrence or dispute, consuming fast food can be a way to divert your mind from handling the situation.

Emotional eating's result is still the same. The feelings that contributed to it don't matter. The emotions come back, even with the guilt of not keeping faith in the weight loss target.

It can then contribute to the unhealthy cycle where our feelings cause us to over-feed, we blame ourselves for not achieving our target, feel discouraged and then feed again. Here are some strategies you can use to regulate emotional eating and bring your weight loss goals back on track.

1. Put the things you want to do in the list and hang it where you can easily see it. You may be so busy caring for others that you don't even know what you enjoy. The more you concentrate on what you want, the more you will feel happy and not eat emotionally.

2. You can use meditation, relaxation, and yoga to relieve stress. Through meditation, you will relax your mind through beautiful words to offer you strength.

3. Avoid boredom: Instead of snacking when you're not hungry, browsing the internet, walking, listening to music, playing with kids, or just reading.

4. When you find it hard to avoid sweet and convenient foods, don't eat them where you can easily access them. Stop going to the grocery store when the feelings aren't entirely controlled.

5. Spoil yourself once in a while and add variety to curb your cravings. If you consume too many calories, you may eat too many of the same stuff while avoiding the treatments you enjoy. It increases your cravings when emotionally stressed.

6. Eat nutritious snacks: eat fresh fruits, vegetables (apple, carrot, cucumber), or sugar-free, butter-free popcorn between meals: Low-calorie, low-fat snacks.

You want to lose weight because you love yourself and your body. So, if you break the law, forgive yourself and continue the next day. Benefit from the mistake and handle your potential weight better. If you are happy to make positive changes in your eating habit, you will finally reach your ideal weight.

Chapter 24 How to Eat Right with The Help of Meditation

- Eat fruits

When was the last time you went to the market intending to buy fruits specifically? You find that we purchase all other types of food, but we barely think of buying fruits. The good thing about fruits is that they are healthy, and they have plenty of nutritional benefits. If you are the type of person that loves sweet things, fruits can act as a suitable replacement. When consumed, they add value to your body and can prevent you from acquiring some diseases. Fruits also contain some minerals that are essential to your body. Now the question we have at the moment is how mediation will help you in taking the fruits. One of the benefits of meditating is that it allows you to differentiate between right and wrong. Eating fruits is beneficial to your body, and hence it is an excellent move to take.

- Avoid processed foods

Currently, we are having a lot of processed foods. The food industry has been one of the fastest-growing industries. As the industry expands, the market becomes competitive, and more people join the industry. We are introducing new foods to the market as companies look forward to growing and gaining recognition. One of the common factors among all the companies is that they aim at pleasing the consumers. After carefully studying the target market, they know what each individual requires, which helps them produce their various items. If they target a market with low purchasing power, they make products that are cheap and enticing. Some of the processed foods made by such companies contain many chemicals and have harmful effects on the individual. You find that such foods are not helpful and only result in harm. These are the types of foods that we need to avoid if we wish to have good health. One of the things that you require for you to avoid such foods is discipline. It allows you to make the right decisions regarding what you consume, and you only take in what is helpful.

- Avoid carbohydrates

In every meal that you take, you only require a small portion of carbohydrates. In most cases, we do the contrary and have the most considerable percentage of our feed as a carbohydrate. When we go to this, our body receives more than it can utilize. One of the primary purposes of consuming carbohydrates is that they provide us with energy. When they are consumed in excess, not all can be used to provide power. The quantity can be turned into fatty tissues, and one ends up adding some weight.

It is better to avoid taking large amounts of carbohydrates because, in some cases, they can result in some diseases like cardiovascular diseases. Ensure that you only take the recommended portions. You also find that some of these foods, like bread, contain certain addictive substances. In the process, all you want to do is keep wishing to take more. As a result, you take up more than your body needs, and the excess does not benefit it in any. Mediation can help you attain some self-control. You get to eat the amount of food that your body requires.

- Eating the recommended portion of food

Eating right can mean taking the amount of food that one needs. You find that certain chronic eating disorders prevent us from eating as we should. An individual with bulimia tends to consume more food than the required portion. Various factors can cause an individual to do so. For instance, they might be struggling with low self-esteem due to how they look. Some petite individuals wish they were a little bit bigger. As a result of their esteem issues, they consume more than the required amount of food. They have a specific belief that if they eat a lot, they will get to the size they want. Sadly, that is not always the case. At times their body experiences no change, which can cause an individual to be frustrated. The same applies to eating less than the required amount of food. Skipping some meals is not good. You end up causing more harm to your body when you should be taking proper care of it. The best thing to do is to ensure that you take the recommended amount. It ensures that you stay healthy and fit. With the aid of mediation, you can maintain focus.

- Consuming plant-based meals

Everyone should turn to eat vegetables. Plant-based meals contain nutrients that are helpful to our bodies. Some minerals are present to ensure that our bodies function and normal body processes are being conducted well. The nutrients are effective in ensuring that we maintain good health by providing minerals that prevent certain diseases. Some of these minerals help in boosting the various metabolic processes occurring in our bodies. In case you have not been consuming plant-based meals, you have been missing a lot. Plant-based meals are also effective in weight loss.

They ensure that we take only the right food portion that is helpful to our bodies. When most people want to start a weight loss journey, the immediate solution is talking plant-based meals. They have proven to be beneficial in that journey and process. In the past, people used to live long and were healthy because of consuming such diets. At this time, people would eat what they planted or what they hunted. They ate right and led healthy life. One needs some discipline for them to eat plant-based meals.

- Eat lightly cooked food

When we overcook meals, they do not have nutritional benefits to our bodies. You find that all the nutrients that were present are lost in the process. As you consume that food, it is not helpful to your body. Foods are beneficial when raw or when lightly cooked. Not everyone might manage to eat the foods when they are in this state. One needs a certain level of discipline to cook their food and consume it in that state lightly. At times you find that it is easier to consume food when fully cooked, especially with the taste that comes with it. You want to eat something sweet and something that you can easily chew. The problem with such desires is that the food will not help you in any way. At times you are torn between enjoying your meal or eating right. The two are difficult choices to choose from, and you may find yourself opting to enjoy your meal. Eating healthy can be fun, only if you tune your mind into it. Meditation will help you maintain focus, and you will efficiently accomplish the goals that you have set.

- Reduce your sugar intake

Sugars are sweet and enticing. They make you want to eat more, and you simply cannot have enough of them. At times you crave to eat something sweet to your taste buds. The problem is the effect that these sugars have on your body. You find that when you consume them in excess, they cannot be utilized by the body. Instead of being converted into energy, they are converted into fats. When this happens, it can result in further complications to your body. We have some diseases such as diabetes that result from consuming excessive sugars. We also have some challenges, such as tooth problems that result from consuming sugars.

At times they can be addictive, and all we wish to do is take more of them. However, with the proper discipline, we can regulate our sugar consumption. You can decide that you will be taking only a certain amount of sugars in a day. Meditation allows you to be focused on what you do. In this case, your focus is on regulating the number of sugars that you take. With this, you get to consume that which is necessary. In the end, it ensures that you have good health and that your body is in the right shape

- Avoid overeating

Overeating is a bad eating habit that everyone should avoid. In overeating, one gets to add extra weight, and it has some harmful effects on their body. Mindful eating is essential in ensuring that we maintain good health. An individual's ability to focus can help them know when they are full. Different foods have different food components. Some foods will make you feel full at a fast rate than others will. You can analyze how your body feels after eating certain types of foods and know the effect of each food. This analysis helps you determine the portion that you should consume depending on the kind of food involved. As a result, you make better and more informed decisions about what you consume and watch the quantity you take. To effectively follow this, one requires self-control that ensures they stick to the plan. It may appear like a challenging thing to accomplish, but it is possible with the help of meditation. You only need to tune your mind into consuming that which is necessary.

Chapter 25 Background Information for Weight Loss

You may find yourself developing some habits without knowing. The same applies to creating excellent health practices. Your daily routines and choices explain your current conditions. Stop complaining; do focus on your habits a remember your preferences will define who you will be. Albert Einstein goes on to say, "we cannot solve our problems with the same thinking we used when we created them." Step out of your bubble a given structure for the desired outcome. Really the most challenging part is starting, and you've already done that, and it will only get more accessible and more natural the more you participate and the more you take an active role in this journey.

Consider habits development as elaborated in the story of a Miller and a camel on a winter day. It was freezing outside, and while the miller was asleep, he was awakened by some noise on the door. Upon opening his eyes, he heard the voice of a camel complaining that it was cold outside and was requesting to warm his nose inside. Miller agreed that he was only to insert the nozzle. A little later, the camel put his forehead, neck, and other parts of the body than the whole-body bit by bit until he started destroying things inside. He started walking in the house, stumbling on anything on its way. When the miller ordered the camel to move out, he boasted that he was comfortable inside and would not leave. The camel went further to tell the miller that he could leave at his pleasure. The same goes for a habit that comes knocking about and taking over.

Maybe you started out smoking your first cigarette, thinking it was disgusting, and then years go by, and you have a nasty habit. Well, bad habits can sneak in, but the same philosophy can apply to ethical practices. Just take it bit by bit and step by step, and before you know it, you have healthy habits in your life. There are so many challenges to healthy eating. You have to be willing to have an open mind and reset your thinking on food.

It is cheaper to develop new habits; effort is the primary requirement, but not that much. When you have trained yourself new patterns, train on it every day for some time, after which it will be automatic.

We can relate that situation to a football club Coash who participates in rigorous training with his players while awaiting the match. They practice new skills and moves. When match day arrives, the coach sits with the substitutes while watching the players playing from the line. Players play as per the learned skills and moves. Apply the required effort to actualize your goal.

While storying with your workmates, tell them how you drink 3 to four glasses of water every day, the same as tea. That looks strict. At heart, you know how your consumption of water and team is reduced while at home. It is a self-discipline that calls for the establishment of solid foundations. Efforts adopted are less.

Apply Core solutions

Recognize and face the challenges of healthy eating and develop new habits. Like a logger trying to clear a log, identify the critical side of each situation. The well-experienced logger will try to identify essential joints by climbing up then doing the clearing.

A less experienced logger would start by the edge. Both methods produce expected results, but one way saves more time and uses less energy than the other. All our problems have strategic points. How about when we identify critical logs to healthy eating and offer some solutions. First, log jam how you were brought up. You may have been forced as a child to eat vegetables and see them as something undesirable, and you built a perception that plants don't taste good. Another log jam is stress—so much pressure.

We live in a world full of pressure where time matters in all our undertakings, troubled life, and our bodies pay most of the price. You have many choices to pick from. If you are a lover of fast food, you need to stop. Fast foods are addictive, and we highly depend on them due to their positive attitude towards them. We are obsessed with them such that we cannot live a day without consuming them. When you eat something wrong for you, and you say you don't care. Your thoughts and focus are totally on how delicious and enjoyable it is to be eating the food that you're eating, regardless of how unhealthy it is, and then you have guilt about how those pounds are going on rather than coming off.

Such thoughts occur even when taking tasty food. We may find ourselves eating some food which in reality we know are very dangerous to our health. Chip is a prime example. An individual from a diet class may feel hungry on her way back home and decide to a branch by a fast food joint for some plates of chips. Despite several cautions on the dangers of chips from class lessons, she chooses to eat chips — what a radical idea. Most people have mental disorders making it difficult to stop taking some food even though we understand their repercussions on our bodies. i.e., eating chips. An article on this topic claims that most food companies work hard at night to make fast food more addictive.

According to Howard Moskovitz, a consultant in the junk food industry, they put more flavor on junk food to make you come back for more. If the food tastes too good, then we'd have what's called a sensory-specific Satia T then we wouldn't want anymore. So, companies have to find just the right balance of flavors. So, there's not too much or too little. All they do is balance the flavors. That balance is called Bliss point.

According to Steven Weatherly, an expert in junk food, Cheetos are the core source of pleasure. They are the specific type of food manufactured by big companies to satisfy you and not add any health benefit to your body. They are designed so that it melts in your mouth when you start eating them, making them feel tasty and impressive. They are made to make you go for more. A friend was once a diet, and her boyfriend brought home Cheetos. Yes, she said no. She ended up just having one, and before she knew it, she knew almost the whole thing. Now we understand why the following log in our way may think we don't like healthy food. Perhaps you don't like healthy food. You want foods that excite your palate to feel alive, be closer to something exciting, but you will not be satisfied.

You'll not reach the maximum point, and perhaps you will not know what to do. Normalizing bad habits make us feel comfortable in our negative thoughts. When you do one negative thing, the effects widely spread. Self-indulgence keeps us wrapped up in this safe place and keeps us inside of ourselves and absorbed by negative thoughts. You know you do one thing poorly or negatively; it trickles into other areas. It leaves you feeling bad, and you do short to feel better just for the short term, such as impossible diets that you can't keep up with, and then you, you feel worse and worse about yourself and you, you go overboard when you can't keep up. It's a vicious cycle. The primary method of overcoming these critical logs is to push the reset button immediately. It might not be easy; strive as much as you can by having an open mind and a positive attitude in the future.

Explore various flavors even if you don't like them. Michael's sister has a negative attitude towards blueberries. Since her childhood, she had not consumed any and kept telling stories that had no connection to the blueberries' taste. One day Michael made her taste the blueberry, and she loved it. Test your assumptions; test your opinions because you don't know where they came from; such an assumption may be baseless.

Despite her premise on blueberries being messy, she made a try, and she ended up loving it. Open your mind to new ideas. Remember the story of the coy and to keep figuratively throwing yourself in more significant environments, you will stretch out and grow in size. Adopt an attitude of success, stop fetus thinking, and know that your thoughts, perceptions, and behaviors can change. Why not start to look forward to fruits and vegetables, however crazy they sound? You were not born with thoughts you possess today; they are a construct of your mind. They can be challenged.

The following solution calls for changing one's health. Saying a big NO and breaking a cycle is all you need — cutting out indulgence.

Commit yourself daily, and you'll find it easier to overcome the notion of food industries that want you to be addicted to their food. The third is growth towards what you want and the freedom you desire. This step calls for exceptional consistency. Make your bold step a pattern. This pattern will develop into the desired habit. Unpack your true self through spiritual faith and meditative silence. Strive to become better. Look inside; stop looking for solutions on the outside. Make additional efforts like being more helpful to those that are happy and caring for those that are needy, consistently reach for truth, grace, and peace in your day. Take caution on being a man of the people, and you may be living a fishy life. Finally, systems generate autonomy. We will be creating a plan together by planning, keeping it simple, embracing balance in your life, and accomplishing these solutions and your goals by following the system to help you prioritize and reinforce consistency in your life.

The best solution to weight loss is a healthy diet and an active body. There could be a reason why doing these two is a problem from your side. The pathway will make the process more holistic and more fun. It may not be your answer, but you must get something from it.

Chapter 26 The Final Weight Loss Puzzle

We can all be thin when we choose to, but most of us have been brainwashed with weight-loss companies and diets that tend to ignore our bodies and instead follow medical establishments blindly. Our bodies are also wiser than the several varieties of diets in the market. However, with diverse information reporting how unhealthy foods will affect our weight, we have turned deaf ears to what the body communicates. That is why this book is dedicated to revealing to you the puzzle you need to change your lifestyle forever.

The secret to becoming naturally thin is to follow the four basic rules of life simply. The rules will guide you on when to eat, how to eat, what to eat, and how much you need to eat to avoid weight gain. These habits will enable you to eat whatever you crave and ensure that you have the healthiest body.

Eat Only When You Are Hungry

When you choose to starve your body, you might begin to lose weight but only for a short time. The body will react immediately by slowing down the metabolism process to ensure that enough fats are stored for the body. It is usually aimed at allowing the body to survive for a more extended period until it refeeds.

As soon as you begin eating, the boy will naturally store up all the food as a way of preparing itself for the subsequent starvation. It means that when you constantly eat after a period of starving, all the food will be stored in fats, resulting in weight gain.

Additionally, some people may find themselves overeating once they move beyond a period of starvation. The body is usually hungry, and it is always difficult to control how much one eats, causing an influx in the number of calories that the body can contain. In such a case, you may find yourself gaining back all the weight you gained during starvation but also end up gaining even more.

So, the bottom line is when you are hungry, you should EAT without hesitation.

Stop Eating When You Are Full

Another important step towards attaining a slim body is always to stop eating when you feel full. One of the ways to know when you are full is to put your spoon or fork down between your bites. The automatic cycle of hand-to-mouth as people eat may cause overfeeding. Once you take a bite, give your spoon or fork rest to tune into your body's cues. You will be able to tell when you are full and satisfied.

An important tip to always stop eating when feeling full is turning off any distractions while eating. Studies have shown that people tend to eat 14 times more when they watch TV. It is associated with a lack of mindful eating that makes us unable to control our food intake.

Eat Only What You Crave

The ongoing love-hate relationship we have with food, eating what you want, not what you think you should, sounds like an imaginary piece of cake. We often forget that eating is one of life's simplest pleasures. Deprivation of certain foods makes them all the more attractive to you. Eating what you want creates a balanced relationship with all foods. Most diabetics when asked, what food they miss the most, are those restricted by the doctors, that is, salts, sugar (sweetened food), and white grubs. It is because their relationship with these foods created tension that upset the balance. Listening to your body releases you from the guilt and anxiety from not following a strict dietary plan.

Enjoying food is essential because then you can listen to it when you have had enough. Provided you are hungry, you are free to eat whatever you want and thoroughly enjoy it. Trust your gut because you are no longer what you eat but why you eat. The reasons you eat make a world of difference in informing your meal decisions; when to eat, what to eat, and when to stop. A few elements make food pleasurable: smell, taste, temperature, substance, presentation, and texture. When you crave a cheesy, warm, savory meal, a crispy, cold salad will not do the trick. You will not receive the same satisfaction from it as much as you expected with the warm meal.

Denying yourself foods that you like often leads to over-eating when you do get the chance to eat them, as well as the foods you are currently "permitted" to eat. The reason for this is that you wind up looking for satisfaction elsewhere. The pleasure you expect to feel with certain foods is not easily substituted with different foods. Additionally, eating meals you do not like would lead you to eat quickly to finish, which is not necessarily a responsible thing to do. Eating slowly helps you listen to when you become full.

When you enjoy your food, the following happens:

•   You digest your food better. Your gastrointestinal system relaxes, releasing more digestive juices. When you eat something with guilt, your body is under stress, and that tension puts a strain on the digestive tract causing it to be that much slower and triggering gut issues like bloating.

•   You will be satisfied with less.

•   You absorb more nutrients. When you enjoy the food, absorption of nutrients takes effect mainly because the entire digestive tract is working at optimum capacity.

We are fully aware of our nutritional needs. Most people worry that if they always gave in to their cravings, they might never make healthy decisions. The contrary is true. Your body is always asking for different things at different times of the day and through the weeks. Any food that does not cause you pleasure should not form any part of your meal.

Eat Consciously and Enjoy Every Bite You Make

Eating consciously involves mindfulness with every food you buy, prepare, serve, and consume. Most people eat far too quickly to induce the feel-good hormone that is discharged with feelings of pleasure. Eating fast then makes you overlook the signs of satisfaction that your body is hinting at you, and you end up stretching out your stomach and putting on weight. The same pleasure you chased fleetingly disappears, and the guilt takes hold. To alleviate the responsibility, you crave food, and the vicious cycle continues.

Mindfulness provides a balance between overeating and undereating while making you consciously aware of every bite and the sensations that accompany it. It is impossible to do something unless you know exactly what you are doing. That said, it is more important to feed your hunger than to feed your face. Unconsciously gulping down food like a barn animal brings about unwanted physical, psychological, and emotional concerns.

To reclaim your consciousness when eating:

• Start with your grocery shopping. Make sure you only purchase the foods you thoroughly enjoy.

• Exercise regular self-observation and be compassionate to yourself in case you catch yourself slipping.

• Allocate time to meals. Take about thirty minutes to an hour out of your day to sit down and enjoy your food.

• Avoid multitasking and distractions during meal times. Avoid eating in front of the fridge or the Tv. Sit down with your food as the only thing in front of you and engage your senses.

• Always serve your meal on a plate or a bowl. Avoid eating from the packaging.

• Take small bites and chew thoroughly while engaged in every mouthful

The focus would be to shift your mind from just thinking about food to taking yourself on an Epicurious journey. Eating consciously leads to emotional health, along with:

• Reducing stress on the body and the mind

• Eating consciously, according to researchers, helps you reach your optimal weight by cutting the excessive eating

• Healthy blood sugar levels

- Improved relationship with food

Exercising mindfulness in food as well as life generally leads you to do the right things properly. Food is food. There is no "good" nor "bad" (unless it is inedible), and at this point, it fails to qualify as food. When we remove the stigma associated with food cravings, we become liberated and begin to enjoy our experiences with food fully. Mindful eating might be new to Western culture, but it has been a tried and tested technique in Asian culture over a long period.

When our limiting inner dialogue on food no longer guides us, we can cultivate new thoughts based on our conscious eating- freed from the shackles of deprivation of certain types of food. Our approach to food and eating experiences becomes something to which we can look forward. Awareness with food gives a pause allowing us to consider our impulses and reactions from time to time. To unlock mindfulness eating, ask yourself how you relate to food and be frank with yourself. It is also noteworthy to note that not all people have the same relationship dynamic with food.

Chapter 27 Tips for Great and Healthy Living

The ideal approach to accomplish better wellbeing is to change your way of life. It's tied in with causing a change from the nourishments you eat to the exercises you do in your regular day-to-day existence. You can begin by staying away from lousy nourishments, slick and handled food sources since they will include more pounds into your body just as you start setting aside some effort to work out.

It will empower you to have a better capacity to burn calories, which will help you consume more fats just as get your body fit as a fiddle. It is only something you can do to remain sound. To get more direction, simply read on as right now, we share with you tips on how you can begin your way towards a more useful life and you! Appreciate!

1. Sleep for at any rate of 8 hours every night.

Having enough rest is part of the most significant activities to improve and keep up your wellbeing. It can make you increasingly vigorous the following day, besides how it can likewise forestall binge eating. All the more significantly, it is additionally perhaps the ideal approach to prevent diseases since it toughens your insusceptible framework.

2. Wash your hands as often as possible.

Washing your hands the same number of times as you can for the entire day is perhaps the most ideal approach to forestall diseases. It ought to be finished with running water and a decent antibacterial cleanser. What's more, washing ought to be accomplished for, in any event, 20 seconds, to guarantee that it is liberated from any malady disease germs.

3. Never skip breakfast.

If your objectives are to get more benefits and to abstain from putting on an excessive amount of weight, at that point, skipping breakfast ought to be the keep going thing on your mind. Breakfast is the critical meal of the day. The feed can prop you up all consistently. If you skip it, odds are, you will put on weight because of binge eating and limited capacity to burn calories.

4. Drink, at any rate, eight glasses of water every day.

Water can help your body in flushing out poisons. Besides that, it can likewise guarantee that you are appropriately hydrated. Besides, drinking water can also help in stifling your hunger, which results in a fitter you. In this manner, make sure that you drink at any rate eight glasses of water each day to keep up your wellbeing.

5. Limit espresso consumption.

Espresso can influence the nature of your absorption, which is why it ought not to be drilled all the time. A great many people drink various cups of espresso every day. To get more benefits, it is ideal for chopping it down to only one container for each day or make drinking espresso a trivial thing.

6. Purchase a littler plate to either chop down your weight or to look after it.

Decreasing the measure of nourishments that you eat in every meal can emotionally impact keeping up or shedding pounds. Something you can accomplish for it is buying a little plate, which is for your utilization. With a bit of dish, you can fool yourself into eating littler segments, which would give you bunches of medical advantages over the long haul.

7. Try not to eat whatever isn't on your plate.

Acquire control over the measure of nourishment you eat every day; it is ideal to abstain from eating food that isn't on your plate. There are many occasions when you might need to get a bunch of peanuts out of the holder or take a soup sample out of the bowl with a spoon. If you keep on doing this, at that point, you include more calories into your body without knowing it.

8. Eat more slowly.

Eating quick is probably the ideal way if you need to put on more weight. Like this, you are doing something contrary to that, which can lose an abundance of pounds of weight. In this way, the time has come to make the most of your meals more by eating more slowly. At the point when you eat more slowly, you can stifle your craving, and it can likewise cause you to feel full, regardless of whether you have not expended a lot of nourishments yet after a specific timeframe.

9. Be sound emotionally.

Unlike a few people may accept, your feelings likewise assume an incredible job regarding your well-being. In this manner, it is ideal for overseeing it, attempting to forestall blowing up, and consistently attempting to have an uplifting viewpoint of life. At the point when you do this, you can get more settled in most testing circumstances.

10. Think positive.

A few people may not trust it, yet your mind can influence your wellbeing in specific manners. For instance, if you generally imagine that you are becoming ill, at that point, it will build your odds of getting influenced by an ailment. Then again, if you believe that you are stable, at that point, you become increasingly dynamic, and it would likewise support your insusceptible framework.

11. Dodge popular fashion diets.

Most craze diets are diet programs, which are intended to cause individuals to get more fit quickly. By and large, these projects can include causing the individual to experience starvation, resulting in a quicker rate of getting more fit. In any case, because of the way that it has been accomplished, you can restore the weight in merely an issue of weeks, and you may even get heavier than when you formerly began with it.

12. A brisk stroll for 3 to multiple times every week.

Energetic strolling is a movement that you can appreciate with your loved ones. It can help in boosting your digestion, which can result in weight loss. Besides that, it can likewise take care of business, your hips, bottom, just as your legs. Intend to energetic stroll for at any rate 20 minutes in 3 to 4 times each week, to pick up the advantages from it.

13. Exploit practice recordings.

If you are the sort of individual, who wouldn't like to invest energy in driving to find a right pace rec center, at that point, remind yourself that there are practice recordings that you can exploit. These recordings can be played at the solaces of your home whenever you need them. You should simply follow the schedules that appeared in it and appreciate them.

14. Play with your children all the more frequently

Children are so lively, and we regularly wonder why. Be that as it may, if you play with them, you can help your vitality level too. It can result in a higher metabolic rate. In this manner, it can assist you with consuming more fats and calories. Besides, doing it frequently can likewise give you an approach to bond with them more.

15. Drink a glass of water when you wake up.

Drinking a glass of water after awakening offers a ton of medical advantages. For one, it gets your framework working, which can support up your vitality level. What's more, it can likewise help in purging your assemblage of poisons that have been aggregated for a long while.

16. Sharing is something that you ought not to do in ensuring your wellbeing.

With regards to your wellbeing, sharing ought not to be finished. It relates to sharing your things with different people, such as hankies, toothbrushes, nail cutters, and such. The facts demonstrate that sharing is acceptable. However, this ought not to be watched about your things.

17. Mind your pets.

A few people don't know that there are sure ailments, which can be transmitted from creature to people. Along these lines, if you have pets, at that point, ensure that they are given their suggested inoculations. What's more, you ought to likewise make sure that they are appropriately prepped, with the goal that they are liberated from ticks and bugs that may also convey germs.

18. Try not to confound ache to hunger.

There are times when we open up our coolers to get a bite, in any event, when our body is aching for water. It is because we tend to decipher thirst as appetite. Consequently, if you want to eat in any event, when you have quite recently had your meal, at that point, attempt to drink a glass of water. By and large, you will feel fulfilled due to it, particularly since you were dehydrated in any case.

19. Maintain a strategic distance from prepared nourishments as much as you can.

Handled nourishments like franks, burgers, French fries, and such don't contain enough supplements to furnish your body with what it needs. Besides that, they are likewise topped off with a ton of artificial flavorings, which can make your body amass bunches of poisons. Therefore, it is ideal to evade them for as much as you can. Staying away from them can help forestall maladies, besides how it would likewise help make you more beneficial.

20. Eat nourishments that are high in fiber content.

If one of your wellbeing objectives is to shed a couple of pounds, at that point load up on fiber, fiber draws out the absorption procedure, which implies that it can cause you to feel full more. At the point when that occurs, you usually are stifling your hunger. Besides that, fiber can likewise help in freeing your assortment of waste.

21. Cut down your utilization of carbonated sodas.

Carbonated sodas are stacked with a great deal of sugar, which can make you put on weight, and it can even build your odds of getting diabetic. A few people who are partial to drinking such refreshments incline toward diet ones since they guarantee to contain lesser sugar measures. Be that as it may, such beverages are stacked with aspartame, which can cause heaps of medical problems over the long haul.

22. Utilize the stairs rather than the lift.

At whatever point you report to your office, make it likely to utilize the stairs rather than the lift. It can offer an original route for you to consume more fats and calories. It is a type of activity, which can fortify your leg muscles, and it is a decent option in contrast to running or lively strolling.

23. Eat more organic products.

Organic products are stacked with natural nutrients and dampness to keep you feeling better. It is perhaps the ideal approach to forestall ailments and blockage. Most organic products additionally contain chemicals that help your body engross the supplements offered by the nourishments you eat.

Chapter 28 Getting Off the Roller Coaster

Diet systems remain quiet about the fact they thrive on failure. Many people who diet lose weight initially, but statistics show that the vast majority — more than 80%—won it back in five years, and others saw it for decades. And for reasons that scientists are only beginning to understand, many people who lose weight on a diet get it all back, and then some, ending up heavier and less balanced than people who never died first.

Dieting psychology can be the most harmful of all, and it affects us all—dieters and non-dieters alike. Diet-related thought patterns have been part of our social environment for decades and are weakening the eating habits of us all. What's more, the entire notion of progress has been corrupted by food culture and the diet industry. The approach to changing our behaviors through just-do-it, power-through-it, all-or-nothing, with encouragement from outside oneself, lacks the secret to real, positive change: You. To build a healthier relationship with food and your body, you need to recognize the diet mindset for what is a false promise that will set you to fail—and start the process of improving from within.

The Diet Seduction

For decades, many people have tried to lose weight and, not surprisingly, feel disappointed with their lack of success and desperate for something that works. If you're dealing with weight loss, slogans, and assurances, that may not be realistic, but music to your ears is easy to fall victim to. Stop, you're eating fights now! Eat everything that you want, and never feel hungry! We have a Magic Weight Loss Recipe!

The marketing strategies of diet companies also tap into body insecurity, with promises you'll get your "best body," shed 20 pounds per bikini season, or lose your baby's belly, and great photos of the supposed results. A hallmark of typical diets is the belief that there's a slim, toned, youthful body inside you waiting to break free — that this is, indeed, the real you. They also tend to target particular body parts — for women; it's most often the belly, thighs, or ass. Our bodies naturally store extra fat in these places, and many of us harbor negative feelings.

Not every typical diet is flagrantly reckless. But even the "better" ones, with sound nutritional strategies, appear to fail. It's only the particulars of a particular diet that are problematic — it's the very essence of dieting.

Most organized diet plans have a clear and seductive message: consume those foods in those amounts, and you will lose weight. The underlying premise is that, with hyper-controlled feeding, the cure for out-of-control feeding is to clamp on it. The method has an obvious appeal. When you struggle to consume nutritious food in small quantities, surrendering to an external authority who tells you exactly what to do may sound like a huge relief. Yet dieting can be a practical emphasis yet approach on aspects of life that are too difficult or complex to be discussed (and often even recognized). As their holy grail, people always look to weight loss. If I lose weight, it will work out the rest of my life, the thought goes. In reality, as you learned in exploring your Wheel of Safety, it's always the other way around.

Despite their appeal, depending on an external authority—external motivation—is setting you to fail. Evidence demonstrates, as described above that internal reason is essential for long-term, lasting change in behavior. You don't answer why you're overeating and eating food in the first place when you follow a prescription schedule. Without that crucial insight, reverting to old habits as soon as you follow the rules is normal, even unavoidable. Whatever diet you adopt may momentarily overpower your habits, but at the end of the diet, those habits are alive and well—and always re-emerge with a vengeance. And considering the autopilot aspect of eating — the fact that when you do, there are countless reasons for taking the first bite or not stopping — it is no wonder why.

The Diet Mentality

Diet-related habits of thinking have become the societal standard, and they are particularly harmful in that they hinder positive progress rather than encourage it. From a psychological point of view, many beliefs that people hold about food, diet, weight loss, and our bodies are cognitive distortions—unconscious habits of thought that are not founded on.

Black-and-white thinking (all-or-nothing thinking) is a dominant cognitive illusion that has become part of our cultural zeitgeist. For example, there's good food and poor food; certain things are off-limits, you're either a safe eater or an unhealthy eater, you're either "on the wagon" or off the wagon, you're never supposed to eat after 8 p.m. There are safer options and less healthy choices, and our plan will direct you to the safer ones. But why does it matter you feed, even though you consume good food? If you base your plans on strict guidelines, it is nearly impossible not to violate them at some stage. Catastrophic, a cognitive illusion that frequently follows all-or-nothing, though, arises when you assume that your behavior or inaction would result in catastrophic consequences, as I did not do this morning. I'm never going to get in shape, and therefore I'm going to be overweight forever. Maybe the most omnipresent misconception is the illusion of willpower, the notion that succumbing to unhealthy cravings (or falling off the diet wagon) is a weakness of will and a sign of personal failure. Cultivating willpower is crucial in learning to postpone gratification but believing it's the only thing required in our over-the-top food world is impractical.

The Enemy Within

There's no room for error when you set yourself up with strict, black and white guidelines to abstain entirely from those foods. You are on or off the diet, either. You're off the wagon once you've had the cookie—and that means anything goes. What's the difference between two and twelve cookies? Next week you will continue the sugar ban again — or probably next month.

Here's the worst part: the guilt, embarrassment, and self-criticism resulting from "breaking the rules" that absolutely prevent you from making healthy efforts. It may sound like self-sabotage, but it's very logical in fact: if you realize you're going to be punished for failure, why try? Who needs punishment? In our curriculum, we refer to ourselves as the Inner Critic, the self-critical element. It's a harsh inner voice that focuses on only one part of ourselves—such as a sugar weakness—with a mean heart, without looking at the bigger picture of who we are. The criticism of getting dishes from the Inner Critic causes one to feel worse and have less desire to adjust. If it's so frustrating to our accumulated experience trying to improve our actions, we stop trying. Health psychologists refer to the "abstinence violation effect" spiral of failure-shame-avoidance, which violates rigid rules.

Health Happens "In the Middle"

Unusually, our days go exactly as expected – at work, home, and anywhere between. Our children get sick; we get sick; we get stuck in the traffic; we get bad news about a friend's wellbeing; our supervisor adds a job to our overflowing plate.

The diet mentality is detrimental to weight loss and physical wellbeing; it also runs counter to emotional health. Psychologists use cognitive rigidity to describe thought patterns that are so entrenched that people have difficulty thinking flexibly. Humans are not robots. It's natural to have a hard time implementing a strict plan — whether it's a diet, a "detox," or an effort to give up sugar in cold turkey. In an ever-changing environment, versatility is key to maintaining healthy eating habits.

The entire notion of versatility is frightening for many people who have struggled with their eating habits, bringing to mind an "everything goes" mindset that can do nothing but curb their unhealthy habits. And that preoccupation is genuine. We don't say "anything goes." Having plenty of freedom but no expectations or guidance can leave us wandering in our attempts to make changes — we don't even know where to begin. How then, without being locked into a fixed program, can you make changes?

Behavior-changing progress is most successful when individuals are "in the middle" and not at the extremes. It is crucial to have goals and expectations flexible enough to adjust to changing circumstances, including getting off track, improving your eating habits, and continuing those changes. It runs counter to the mindset of the diet and contrary to "everything goes"—and is sustainable.

Conclusion

There are times that we feel unsatisfied with ourselves. Now and again, we wish to have flawless eyes, impeccable noses, and perfect skin, much the same as others. Do you, in some cases, want to have another person's qualities? For what reasons do we once in a while analyze ourselves? For what reason would we say we aren't accommodated with our appearance? We have heard endlessly that we should adore ourselves, despite our missteps or defects. It incorporates things identified with our character, just as our bodies.

Nonetheless, there are not very many individuals who can acknowledge and be content with themselves. It isn't about not having any desire to change. It is a praiseworthy undertaking when one needs to accomplish or hold their looks or care about looking progressively appealing.

Simultaneously, the vast majority is substantially more essential, more severe with themselves than supported. They are persistently disappointed with themselves and don't find in the mirror what others see. A few young ladies feel a tremendous uneasiness taking a gander at one another, both because they don't care for taking a gander at one another as a rule and because they don't care for what they see. Where do these responses originate from?

What typically happens is that you don't take a gander at yourself; you just observe yourself regarding that perfect of excellence that you have in your mind. It is the place disappointment sneaks in. It has to do with the hypothesis of social showdown. We contrast ourselves and those we think about superior to ourselves; confidence is contrarily influenced. We as a whole have a model in the head, a term of examination that we have worked by taking a gander at long periods of magazines, publicizing, and motion pictures with immaculate Hollywood princesses. The mantra must become one and only one: there is no requirement for me to contrast myself with that model since everyone is an exceptional, liberal example, wealthy in the signs of what I am.

Life would be a lot more straightforward and more joyful on the off chance that we could acknowledge ourselves as we seem to be. Plenty of negative feelings would be discharged; we would have not so much pressure, but rather more of the things that genuinely matter come into seeing. The main concern is, on the off chance that we truly need to change something, we can't do it until we make harmony with the present state. It is an endless loop.

The psyche works, in actuality, in a strange way. If we oppose something, we get a more significant amount of it. All things considered, if we concentrate on what is awful, we strengthen the terrible. What we give the most consideration to as we might suspect that something will materialize.

Everything that originates from you that identifies with you is only yours: your emotions, your voice, your activities, your ears, your thighs, your expectations, and your fears. That is the reason you are one of a kind. Be upbeat that you are unique concerning anybody, that you look how you do and that it is simply you. Begin to feel that it's your own body, not something separate you have to live with.

Do you need your home to be much the same as anybody else's? Or on the other hand, do you love the seemingly insignificant details that convey recollections? Don't you love the air of your chaotic spot after playing with your children? Also, the plain window ornament you realize you ought to supplant, yet which your mother sewed and looks so great? Or, on the other hand, the household item that everybody says you should toss out, yet you demand it?

That is how you should feel about your body. You ought to comprehend that you don't have to contrast it and any other individual's since it's challenging to analyze one-of-a-kind things. Moreover, who figures out what delightful and terrible mean? You should not contrast your body with the big names' ideal-looking bodies because they are balanced with Photoshop and are not as genuine and extraordinary as you.

You're not them. You are neither the nearby young lady who, after three kids, appears as though she did at twenty, nor your companion who you believe is beautiful. You ought to acknowledge your body, yet you should go gaga for it. Do you think like Bonnie? Do you figure nobody could cherish you since you have some additional weight? At that point, ask yourself the accompanying inquiries. Might you be able to experience passionate feelings for somebody just on the off chance that they are impeccable looking? Okay, I genuinely love somebody as a result of their body. I'll go further.

Do we truly cherish flawless-looking individuals? I wager you lean toward your blemished buddy rather than an ideal-looking muscle head. You like the little blame of your significant other, spouse, children, and companions since they have a place with you as well. We love flaws superior to culminations.

Isn't it obvious? We don't quantify individuals dependent on their weight. What's more, if you are content with your body and reality, it will likewise show in your brilliance. In what manner would it be a good idea for you to adore your body?

At the point when you have arrived at your toes, come back to your head once more, to your face, and now, going downhill, simply state to all your body parts, "I love you." Even on the off chance that you feel a little inept about it, don't stop. You will have a unique relationship with your appearance. What's more, coincidentally, we should not overlook it; it is anything but a fortuitous event called external. What's inside is increasingly significant. Be that as it may, what's inside is noticeable outside. So, utilize your internal identity to adore your external, and you will be a lot quieter, more joyful, increasingly fulfilled, and progressively specific.

Set the caution and watch yourself for in any event 40 minutes one after another. Doing so could completely change you. Specialists talk about the pestilence spread of self-perception issue. This severe issue drives us to consider ourselves to be deficient each time we take a gander at our bodies. As indicated by the examination, 90.2% of ladies have a modified picture of themselves and are not happy with their bodies, a reality that has a great deal to do with what we look like in the mirror. The mirror is your new weapon: from adversary to partner yet figuring out how to utilize it in the correct manner (Ferrer, 2015).

Praise yourself. You ought to see yourself as and treat yourself with a similar benevolence and a similar reverence that you would save for those you love. You most likely wouldn't have similar immediate reactions you do to yourself, to someone else. Try not to spare a moment to praise yourself, don't be excessively hard on yourself, and pardon yourself when you commit an error. Please dispose of the contempt you feel for yourself, supplant it with more superior comprehension and appreciation. Glance in the mirror and rehash: "I am alluring. I am certain about myself. I am phenomenal!" Do it routinely, and you'll start to see yourself in a positive light. At the point when you arrive at an objective, be pleased. Glance in the mirror and state, "Extraordinary employment, I'm pleased with myself."

Avoid pessimism. Maintain a strategic distance from individuals who discuss their bodies severely. You chance getting contaminated by their frailties and harping on your deficiencies. Life is concise and significant to be devoured by detesting yourself or searching for every imperfection, mainly when the discernment you have of yourself will, in general, be considerably more fundamental than that of others. On the off chance that an individual begins to condemn their body, could you not engage in their pessimism? Change the subject instead or leave. Wear casual garments that reflect what your identity is. All that you have in the closet should improve your body. Try not to wear awkward garments just to dazzle others. Recollect that the individuals who acknowledge themselves consistently look extraordinary.

Wear excellent, intact articles of clothing to dress the body how you merit. Purchase coordinating briefs and bras, even though you are the just one to see them. You will remind your internal identity that you are doing it only for yourself.

Inquire as to yourself and what they think about your best characteristics. It will assist you with creating yourself and advise you that your body has given you to such an extent. You will most likely be amazed to find what others find excellent about you; you have presumably disregarded them.

References

https://www.amazon.com/Rapid-Natural-Weight-Loss-Hypnosis-Women-ebook/dp/B086KZC7LK/ref=sr_1_68?dchild=1&keywords=RAPID+WEIGHT+LOSS+HYPNOSIS&qid=1590388630&refinements=p_n_feature_nineteen_browse-bin%3A9045887011&rnid=9045886011&s=digital-text&sr=1-68

https://www.amazon.com/Rapid-Weight-Loss-Hypnosis-Affirmations-ebook/dp/B083748GGK/ref=sr_1_1?dchild=1&keywords=RAPID+WEIGHT+LOSS+HYPNOSIS&qid=1590278648&s=digital-text&sr=1-1

https://www.amazon.com/Rapid-Weight-Loss-Hypnosis-Self-Discipline-ebook/dp/B081S5GT2H/ref=sr_1_25?dchild=1&keywords=RAPID+WEIGHT+LOSS+HYPNOSIS&qid=1590312780&s=digital-text&sr=1-25

https://www.amazon.com/Weight-Loss-Hypnosis-Affirmations-Hypnotherapy-ebook/dp/B088TRYXPS/ref=sr_1_2?dchild=1&keywords=RAPID+WEIGHT+LOSS+HYPNOSIS&qid=1590278648&s=digital-text&sr=1-2

https://www.amazon.com/Rapid-Weight-Loss-Hypnosis-Self-Hypnosis-ebook/dp/B087M3PSVP/ref=sr_1_23?dchild=1&keywords=RAPID+WEIGHT+LOSS+HYPNOSIS&qid=1590312780&s=digital-text&sr=1-23

https://www.amazon.com/Rapid-Weight-Loss-Hypnosis-effortlessly-ebook/dp/B083FFQHVC/ref=sr_1_9?dchild=1&keywords=RAPID+WEIGHT+LOSS+HYPNOSIS&qid=1590280229&s=digital-text&sr=1-9

https://www.amazon.com/Meditation-weight-loss-mindfulness-self-esteem-ebook/dp/B084F2PP6T/ref=sr_1_17?crid=2Q8E9D7ZLWAY3&dchild=1&keywords=meditation+for+rapid+weight+loss&qid=1590390466&refinements=p_n_feature_nineteen_browse-bin%3A9045887011&rnid=9045886011&s=digital-text&sprefix=meditation+for+rapid+weight+%2Cdigital-text%2C-1&sr=1-17

https://www.amazon.com/Hypnotic-Gastric-Band-Meditation-Emotional-ebook/dp/B088XSYF9H/ref=sr_1_10?dchild=1&keywords=RAPID+WEIGHT+LOSS+HYPNOSIS&qid=1590280229&s=digital-text&sr=1-10

https://www.amazon.com/Rapid-Weight-Loss-Hypnosis-Self-Hypnonis-ebook/dp/B085N6CL97/ref=sr_1_44?dchild=1&keywords=rapid+weight+loss+hypnosis&qid=1590398107&s=digital-text&sr=1-44

https://www.amazon.com/Rapid-weight-loss-hypnosis-self-hypnosis-ebook/dp/B088RFX5HX/ref=sr_1_7?dchild=1&keywords=RAPID+WEIGHT+LOSS+HYPNOSIS&qid=1590280229&s=digital-text&sr=1-7

https://www.amazon.com/Meditation-Rapid-Weight-Loss-Emotional-
ebook/dp/B0859SQD4W/ref=sr_1_14?crid=2Q8E9D7ZLWAY3&dchi
ld=1&keywords=meditation+for+rapid+weight+loss&qid=159038994
0&refinements=p_n_feature_nineteen_browse-
bin%3A9045887011&rnid=9045886011&s=digital-
text&sprefix=meditation+for+rapid+weight+%2Cdigital-text%2C-
1&sr=1-14

https://www.amazon.com/Hypnotic-Gastric-Band-Meditation-
Emotional-
ebook/dp/B088XSYF9H/ref=sr_1_4?dchild=1&keywords=hypnotic+
gastric+band&qid=1590399350&refinements=p_n_feature_nineteen
_browse-bin%3A9045887011&rnid=9045886011&s=digital-
text&sr=1-4

https://www.amazon.com/Hypnosis-Emotional-Sleeping-Overcome-
Anxiety-
ebook/dp/B083ZZKY7R/ref=sr_1_1?dchild=1&keywords=the+power
+of+guided+meditation+for+weight+loss&qid=1590416504&s=digita
l-text&sr=1-1

https://www.amazon.com/dp/B0893JQQBQ/ref=sr_1_8?dchild=1&
keywords=RAPID+WEIGHT+LOSS+HYPNOSIS&qid=1590280229&
s=digital-text&sr=1-8

https://www.amazon.com/Lose-Weight-Meditation-meditations-
affirmations-
ebook/dp/B083FGF1NK/ref=sr_1_38?dchild=1&keywords=rapid+we
ight+loss+hypnosis&qid=1590398107&s=digital-text&sr=1-38

https://www.amazon.com/Hypnosis-Weight-Loss-Books-Motivation-ebook/dp/B088H8LNHK/ref=sr_1_14?dchild=1&keywords=RAPID+WEIGHT+LOSS+HYPNOSIS&qid=1590280229&s=digital-text&sr=1-14

https://www.amazon.com/Rapid-Weight-Loss-Hypnosis-Women-ebook/dp/B086SVNDQF/ref=sr_1_25?crid=6WJDIRA1E9ZN&dchild=1&keywords=rapid+weight+loss+hypnosis+for+women&qid=1590415980&s=digital-text&sprefix=rapid+weight+loss+hypnosis+for+wom%2Cdigital-text%2C416&sr=1-25

https://www.amazon.com/Rapid-Weight-Loss-Hypnosis-Affirmations-ebook/dp/B088KF7T7D/ref=sr_1_18?dchild=1&keywords=RAPID+WEIGHT+LOSS+HYPNOSIS&qid=1590312780&s=digital-text&sr=1-18

https://www.amazon.com/Weight-Loss-Hypnosis-Women-Affirmations/dp/B086WQJFBM/ref=sr_1_7?crid=33U9NGLZGE3HV&dchild=1&keywords=weight+loss+hypnosis+for+women&qid=1590389705&s=digital-text&sprefix=weight+loss+hypno%2Cdigital-text%2C434&sr=1-7

https://www.amazon.com/Rapid-Weight-Loss-Permanently-Struggling-ebook/dp/B0821VTC29/ref=sr_1_41?dchild=1&keywords=rapid+weight+loss+hypnosis&qid=1590398107&s=dhttps://www.amazon.com/Rapid-Weight-Loss-Permanently-Struggling-ebook/dp/B0821VTC29/ref=sr_1_41?dchild=1&keywords=rapid+weight+loss+hypnosis&qid=1590398107&s=digital-text&sr=1-41igital-text&sr=1-41

https://www.amazon.com/WEIGHT-LOSS-HYPNOSIS-WOMEN-AFFIRMATIONS-ebook/dp/B0881V7RBL/ref=sr_1_27?dchild=1&keywords=RAPID+WEIGHT+LOSS+HYPNOSIS&qid=1590319645&refinements=p_n_feature_nineteen_browse-bin%3A9045887011&rnid=9045886011&s=digital-text&sr=1-27

https://www.amazon.com/EXTREME-WEIGHT-LOSS-HYPNOSIS-RAPID-ebook/dp/B07XL4VD2C/ref=sr_1_23?dchild=1&keywords=RAPID+WEIGHT+LOSS+HYPNOSIS&qid=1590319645&refinements=p_n_feature_nineteen_browse-bin%3A9045887011&rnid=9045886011&s=digital-text&sr=1-23

https://www.amazon.com/Rapid-Weight-Loss-Hypnosis-Affirmations-ebook/dp/B085WYBY9F/ref=sr_1_28?dchild=1&keywords=RAPID+WEIGHT+LOSS+HYPNOSIS&qid=1590312780&s=digital-text&sr=1-28

https://www.amazon.com/Rapid-Weight-Loss-Affirmations-Intermittent-ebook/dp/B085XGSCPF/ref=sr_1_27?dchild=1&keywords=rapid+weight+loss&qid=1590393547&refinements=p_n_feature_nineteen_browse-bin%3A9045887011&rnid=9045886011&s=digital-text&sr=1-27

https://www.amazon.com/Rapid-Weight-Loss-Hypnosis-Affirmations-ebook/dp/B087NW8VWY/ref=sr_1_6?dchild=1&keywords=RAPID+WEIGHT+LOSS+HYPNOSIS&qid=1590316337&s=digital-text&sr=1-6

https://www.amazon.com/RAPID-WEIGHT-LOSS-psychology-
meditation-
ebook/dp/B088LV46K5/ref=sr_1_24?dchild=1&keywords=RAPID+
WEIGHT+LOSS+HYPNOSIS&qid=1590312780&s=digital-text&sr=1-
24

https://www.amazon.com/Rapid-Weight-Loss-Hypnosis-Meditation-
ebook/dp/B0851NMHGK/ref=sr_1_26?crid=6WJDIRA1E9ZN&dchil
d=1&keywords=rapid+weight+loss+hypnosis+for+women&qid=1590
416379&refinements=p_n_feature_nineteen_browse-
bin%3A9045887011&rnid=9045886011&s=digital-
text&sprefix=rapid+weight+loss+hypnosis+for+wom%2Cdigital-
text%2C416&sr=1-26

https://www.amazon.com/RAPID-WEIGHT-LOSS-WOMEN-
AFFIRMATIONS-
ebook/dp/B085PXJQKS/ref=sr_1_66?dchild=1&keywords=RAPID+
WEIGHT+LOSS+HYPNOSIS&qid=1590388630&refinements=p_n_f
eature_nineteen_browse-
bin%3A9045887011&rnid=9045886011&s=digital-text&sr=1-66

☐